PET Imaging of the Head and Neck

Guest Editors

MIN YAO, MD, PhD
PETER F. FAULHABER, MD

PET CLINICS

www.pet.theclinics.com

Consulting Editor
ABASS ALAVI, MD, PhD (Hon), DSc (Hon)

October 2012 • Volume 7 • Number 4

SAUNDERS an imprint of ELSEVIER, Inc.

W.B. SAUNDERS COMPANY
A Division of Elsevier Inc.

1600 John F. Kennedy Boulevard • Suite 1800 • Philadelphia, Pennsylvania 19103-2899

http://www.theclinics.com

PET CLINICS Volume 7, Number 4
October 2012 ISSN 1556-8598, ISBN-13: 978-1-4557-4887-7

Editor: Sarah Barth

PET Clinics (ISSN 1556-8598) is published quarterly by Elsevier Inc., 360 Park Avenue South, New York, NY 10010-1710. Months of issue are January, April, July, and October. Periodicals postage paid at New York, NY, and additional mailing offices. Subscription prices per year are $215.00 (US individuals), $297.00 (US institutions), $110.00 (US students), $244.00 (Canadian individuals), $332.00 (Canadian institutions), $124.00 (Canadian students), $260.00 (foreign individuals), $332.00 (foreign institutions), and $134.00 (foreign students). To receive student and resident rate, orders must be accompanied by name of affiliated institution, date of term, and the signature of program/residency coordinator on institution letterhead. Orders will be billed at individual rate until proof of status is received. Foreign air speed delivery is included in all Clinics subscription prices. All prices are subject to change without notice. POSTMASTER: Send address changes to PET Clinics, Elsevier Health Sciences Division, Subscription Customer Service, 3251 Riverport Lane, Maryland Heights, MO 63043. **Customer Service: 1-800-654-2452 (U.S. and Canada); 314-447-8871 (outside U.S. and Canada). Fax: 314-447-8029. E-mail: journalscustomerservice-usa@elsevier.com (for print support); journalsonlinesupport-usa@elsevier.com (for online support).**

Reprints. For copies of 100 or more of articles in this publication, please contact the Commercial Reprints Department, Elsevier Inc., 360 Park Avenue South, New York, NY 10010-1710. Tel.: 212-633-3812; Fax: 212-462-1935; E-mail: reprints@elsevier.com.

Printed and bound by CPI Group (UK) Ltd, Croydon, CR0 4YY

Transferred to digital print 2012

Contributors

CONSULTING EDITOR

ABASS ALAVI, MD, PhD (Hon), DSc (Hon)
Professor of Radiology, Division of Nuclear
Medicine, University of Pennsylvania School of
Medicine; Department of Radiology, Hospital
of the University of Pennsylvania, Philadelphia,
Pennsylvania

GUEST EDITORS

MIN YAO, MD, PhD
Associate Professor of Radiation Oncology,
Case Western Reserve University; Department
of Radiation Oncology, Director of Head and
Neck Radiation Oncology, Seidman Cancer
Center, University Hospital Case Medical
Center, Cleveland, Ohio

PETER F. FAULHABER, MD
Professor of Radiology, Case Western Reserve
University; Division of Nuclear Medicine,
Director, Clinical PET University Hospital Case
Medical Center, Cleveland, Ohio

AUTHORS

**GERARD ADAMS, BSc(Hons), MBChB,
MRCP, FRCR, FRANZCR**
Division of Cancer Services, Department of
Radiation Oncology, Princess Alexandra
Hospital, Queensland, Australia

ABASS ALAVI, MD, PhD (Hon), DSc (Hon)
Professor of Radiology, Division of Nuclear
Medicine, University of Pennsylvania School of
Medicine; Department of Radiology, Hospital
of the University of Pennsylvania, Philadelphia,
Pennsylvania

SANDIP BASU, MD
Professor, Radiation Medicine Centre (BARC),
Tata Memorial Hospital Annexe, Parel,
Mumbai, India

SIMON K. CHENG, MD, PhD
Associate Professor, Department of Radiation
Oncology, College of Physicians and
Surgeons, Columbia University, New York,
New York

GUIDO A. DAVIDZON, MD
Division of Nuclear Medicine, Stanford
University Medical Center, Stanford, California

PETER F. FAULHABER, MD
Professor of Radiology, Case Western Reserve
University; Division of Nuclear Medicine,
Director, Clinical PET University Hospital Case
Medical Center, Cleveland, Ohio

RYAN T. HUBER, MD
Division of Nuclear Medicine, Department
of Radiology, University Case Medical Center;
Resident, Department of Radiology,
University Hospitals Case Medical Center,
Cleveland, Ohio

ROLAND HUSTINX, MD, PhD
Professor, Division of Nuclear Medicine,
University Hospital of Liège, University of
Liège, Liège, Belgium

KIMBERLY J. KINDER, MD
Department of Otolaryngology–Head and Neck Surgery, University Hospitals Case Medical Center, Case Western Reserve University, Cleveland, Ohio

PIERRE LAVERTU, MD
Department of Otolaryngology–Head and Neck Surgery, University Hospitals Case Medical Center, Case Western Reserve University, Cleveland, Ohio

QUYNH-THU LE, MD
Department of Radiation Oncology, Stanford University, Stanford, California

NANCY Y. LEE, MD
Associate Attending, Department of Radiation Oncology, Memorial Sloan-Kettering Cancer Center, New York, New York

MITCHELL MACHTAY, MD
Professor and Chairman, Department of Radiation Oncology, Seidman Cancer Center, University Hospitals of Cleveland, Case Western Reserve University School of Medicine, Cleveland, Ohio

LINA MEHTA, MD
Division of Nuclear Medicine, Department of Radiology, University Case Medical Center; Associate Professor of Radiology, Associate Dean of Admissions, Case Western Reserve University, Cleveland, Ohio

YUSUF MENDA, MD
Associate Professor, Department of Radiology, University of Iowa, Iowa City, Iowa

CAMILA MOSCI, MD
Division of Nuclear Medicine, Stanford University Medical Center, Stanford, California

SANDRO V. PORCEDDU, MBBS(Hons), FRANZCR, MD
Division of Cancer Services, Department of Radiation Oncology, Princess Alexandra Hospital; Faculty of Health Sciences, School of Medicine, University of Queensland, Brisbane, Queensland, Australia

ANDREW QUON, MD
Division of Nuclear Medicine, Stanford University Medical Center, Stanford, California

FARZAN SIDDIQUI, MD, PhD
Department of Radiation Oncology, Henry Ford Hospital, Detroit, Michigan

JASON SOHN, PhD
Associate Professor, Department of Radiation Oncology, Seidman Cancer Center, University Hospitals of Cleveland, Case Western Reserve University School of Medicine, Cleveland, Ohio

MUAMMER URHAN, MD
Associate Professor, Department of Nuclear Medicine, GATA Haydarpasa Training Hospital, Uskudar, Istanbul, Turkey

TONY J.C. WANG, MD
Associate Professor, Department of Radiation Oncology, College of Physicians and Surgeons, Columbia University, New York, New York

CHARLES WOODS, MD
Department of Radiation Oncology, Seidman Cancer Center, University Hospitals of Cleveland, Case Western Reserve University School of Medicine, Cleveland, Ohio

CHENG-CHIA WU, BS
Department of Radiation Oncology, College of Physicians and Surgeons, Columbia University, New York, New York

MIN YAO, MD, PhD
Associate Professor of Radiation Oncology, Case Western Reserve University; Department of Radiation Oncology, Director of Head and Neck Radiation Oncology, Seidman Cancer Center, University Hospital Case Medical Center, Cleveland, Ohio

Contents

> Each anatomic region of the head and neck has physiologic variations that can mimic a primary tumor or lymph node. Many of these variations can be recognized as reflecting benign lymphoid, salivary, brown fat, and muscular activity. A few artifacts are related to computed tomography (CT) attenuation. A knowledge of tumor types and patterns of lymph node and metastatic spread helps categorize patterns as benign or malignant. The anatomic reference of CT helps solve many pitfalls. A recently introduced instrument, PET/magnetic resonance imaging, will face new pitfalls as its role in oncology is developed.

> Diagnostic imaging plays an important role in the staging, restaging, and treatment monitoring in head and neck cancer (HNC). MR imaging and computed tomography (CT) are the primary imaging modalities for the assessment of this type of tumor; however, they have been proved to be ineffective in some cases. ^{18}F-2-fluoro-2-deoxy-D-glucose (FDG) PET/CT and more recently PET/MR imaging are increasingly becoming a standard part of the management of HNC. The purpose of this article is to discuss the indications and benefits of ^{18}F-FDG PET/CT and PET/MR imaging in the management of patients with HNC.

> This article discusses the role of FDG-PETederived parameters as prognostic indicators in patients with squamous cell carcinoma of the head and neck. The basic underlying biology of FDG-PET scans and the quantitative information that can be derived are discussed. A review of the literature is performed. Potential applications in the management of head and neck cancer and future directions in clinical trials are discussed.

> Radiotherapy plays an important role in the management of head and neck cancer. Intensity-modulated radiotherapy is a highly conformal radiation technique that allows delivery of high-dose of radiation to the tumor and high-risk areas while sparing the normal structure. PET scan is a useful tool in identifying the border of the tumor and small lymph nodes with metastatic disease. Future directions in

dose escalation and the use of PET with new tracers other than 18F-fluoro-deoxy-D-glucose are discussed.

This article summarizes the controversies around surgical management of the neck following definitive chemoradiation. It explains how policies have evolved and how changes in the biology of the disease, effectiveness of treatment, and the assessment of results have contributed to this. The focus of the article is on the use of positron emission tomography (PET) in deciding the appropriate management of the neck following treatment. It summarizes available evidence on the clinical usefulness and cost-effectiveness of PET compared with other available strategies.

Fluorodeoxyglucose PET/CT is a powerful tool for staging head and neck squamous cell carcinomas and nasopharyngeal carcinomas. These tumors consistently display high fluorodeoxyglucose uptake, and the PET results are also valuable in terms of prognosis, whether they are obtained before treatment or after its completion. Tumors of the head and neck present distinct clinical features. Evaluating differences in biology among tumor, inflammation, and normal tissue with high physiologic uptake by performing dual time point imaging or post hoc analysis of tissue heterogeneity may also prove highly valuable, although clear clinical data are lacking at this stage.

PET is commonly used in the evaluation and posttreatment management of head and neck squamous cell carcinoma. Although [18F]fluorodeoxyglucose is the most commonly used radiopharmaceutical, many other radiopharmaceuticals are under investigation to assess particular biologic characteristics such as hypoxia and tumor repopulation. In this review, the authors discuss new PET tracers that allow the biologic profiling of head and neck squamous cell carcinomas, including [18F]fluoromisonidazole, [18F]fluorothymidine, [18F]fluoromethyltyrosine, and epidermal growth factor receptor biomarkers.

This article summarizes selected published studies on the use of FDG-PET and PET/CT in the workup of head and neck carcinoma of unknown primary (HNCUP). It shows that PET is a useful imaging modality in identification of the occult primary tumor and discovery of distant metastases. The results of PET often lead to a change in management in these patients. The limitations of PET in HNCUP are also discussed.

Patients with differentiated thyroid carcinoma usually have a good prognosis; however, up to 40% of them may develop local recurrence. PET scanning has added new information on disease evaluation. The most appropriate indication to fluoro-deoxyglucose (FDG) PET scan is in evaluating patients with high thyroglobulin level when I-131 radioiodine whole-body scans are negative and in patients with medullary thyroid carcinoma when the serum calcitonin level is increased. PET scan is also useful in detecting intrathyroid lesions harboring malignancy when FDG uptake in the thyroid is noted incidentally in patients undergoing PET for another indication.

PET CLINICS

GOAL STATEMENT

The goal of the *PET Clinics* is to keep practicing radiologists and radiology residents up to date with current clinical practice in positron emission tomography by providing timely articles reviewing the state of the art in patient care.

ACCREDITATION

PET Clinics is planned and implemented in accordance with the Essential Areas and Policies of the Accreditation Council for Continuing Medical Education (ACCME) through the joint sponsorship of the University of Virginia School of Medicine and Elsevier. The University of Virginia School of Medicine is accredited by the ACCME to provide continuing medical education for physicians.

The University of Virginia School of Medicine designates this enduring material activity for a maximum of 15 *AMA PRA Category 1 Credit*(s)™ *for each issue,* 60 credits per year. Physicians should only claim credit commensurate with the extent of their participation in the activity.

The American Medical Association has determined that physicians not licensed in the US who participate in this CME enduring material activity are eligible for a maximum of 15 *AMA PRA Category 1 Credit*(s)™ for each issue, 60 credits per year.

Credit can be earned by reading the text material, taking the CME examination online at http://www.theclinics.com/home/cme, and completing the evaluation. After taking the test, you will be required to review any and all incorrect answers. Following completion of the test and evaluation, your credit will be awarded and you may print your certificate.

FACULTY DISCLOSURE/CONFLICT OF INTEREST

The University of Virginia School of Medicine, as an ACCME accredited provider, endorses and strives to comply with the Accreditation Council for Continuing Medical Education (ACCME) Standards of Commercial Support, Commonwealth of Virginia statutes, University of Virginia policies and procedures, and associated federal and private regulations and guidelines on the need for disclosure and monitoring of proprietary and financial interests that may affect the scientific integrity and balance of content delivered in continuing medical education activities under our auspices.

The University of Virginia School of Medicine requires that all CME activities accredited through this institution be developed independently and be scientifically rigorous, balanced and objective in the presentation/discussion of its content, theories and practices.

All authors/editors participating in an accredited CME activity are expected to disclose to the readers relevant financial relationships with commercial entities occurring within the past 12 months (such as grants or research support, employee, consultant, stock holder, member of speakers bureau, etc.). The University of Virginia School of Medicine will employ appropriate mechanisms to resolve potential conflicts of interest to maintain the standards of fair and balanced education to the reader. Questions about specific strategies can be directed to the Office of Continuing Medical Education, University of Virginia School of Medicine, Charlottesville, Virginia.

The faculty and staff of the University of Virginia Office of Continuing Medical Education have no financial affiliations to disclose.

The authors/editors listed below have identified no professional or financial affiliations for themselves or their spouse/ partner:

Gerard Adams, BSc(Hons), MBChB, MRCP, FRCR, FRANZCR; Abass Alavi, MD, PhD (Hon), DSc (Hon) (Consulting Editor); Sandip Basu, MD; Adrianne Brigido, (Acquisitions Editor); Simon K. Cheng, MD, PhD; Guido A. Davidzon, MD; Ryan T. Huber, MD; Roland Hustinx, PhD, MD; Kimberly J. Kinder, MD; Pierre Lavertu, MD; Nancy Y. Lee, MD; Mitchell Machtay, MD; Lina Mehta, MD; Camila Mosci, MD; Sandro V. Porceddu, MBBS(Hons), FRANZCR, MD; Patrice Rehm, MD (Test Editor); Farzan Siddiqui, MD, PhD; Jason Sohn, PhD; Muammer Urhan, MD; Tony J.C. Wang, MD; Charles Woods, MD; Cheng-Chia Wu, BS; and Min Yao, MD, PhD (Guest Editor).

The authors/editors listed below identified the following professional or financial affiliations for themselves or their spouse/partner:

Peter Faulhaber, MD (Guest Editor) receives research support and is on the Speakers' Bureau for Philips Medical, and is a consultant for MIM Software.
Quynh-Thu Le, MD receives research support from Varian, GSK, and Amgen.
Yusef Menda, MD receives research support from Siemens Medical Solutions.
Andrew Quon, MD is on the Speakers' Bureau for Eli Lilly.

Disclosure of Discussion of Non-FDA Approved Uses for Pharmaceutical Products and/or Medical Devices.

The University of Virginia School of Medicine, as an ACCME provider, requires that all faculty presenters identify and disclose any off-label uses for pharmaceutical and medical device products. The University of Virginia School of Medicine recommends that each physician fully review all the available data on new products or procedures prior to clinical use.

TO ENROLL

To enroll in the PET Clinics Continuing Medical Education program, call customer service at 1-800-654-2452 or visit us online at www.theclinics.com/home/cme**. The CME program is available to subscribers for an additional fee of $196.00.**

Preface

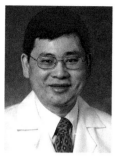
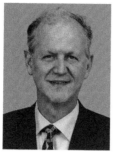

Min Yao, MD, PhD   Peter F. Faulhaber, MD
Guest Editors

FDG-PET is one of the most significant oncologic imaging developments in the last few years. In a relatively short period of time FDG-PET has changed the way we image cancer. One of the reasons for its popularity is its noninvasive nature and ability to demonstrate function rather than just form. Its use has increased our ability to more accurately and noninvasively diagnose and stage malignancies, to evaluate response to therapies, to better guide biopsies and other interventions, and to noninvasively follow patients for recurrences. In addition, recent studies have shown cost savings and changes in treatment regimens based on FDG-PET findings. One of the limitations of FDG, a glucose analog, is its low specificity and a limitation of FDG-PET itself is that of poor anatomic definition; both of these issues have been overcome, or at least mitigated, with the introduction of PET/CT. PET/CT has improved the specificity and accuracy of FDG-PET in initial and subsequent treatment evaluation.[1,2] The confidence of the radiologist in interpreting the study is increased as well with the combined modality.

This issue of the *PET Clinics* will discuss how FDG-PET/CT is becoming the modality of choice not only for staging and restaging of head and neck cancer but also for therapy monitoring, patient prognosis, and radiation therapy planning. The issue begins with how a structured report of an FDG-PET/CT scan based on the tumor, nodes, metastases (TNM) system is the entry point for the patient in the treatment plan. Discussion moves on to how staging can be further advanced by adding MRI as an adjunct to PET/CT in the patient assessment. Then, once a treatment plan such as radiation therapy has been chosen,

PET/CT improves the accuracy of the planning process. New ways of assessing patient prognosis with PET/CT are addressed, including SUV and beyond. The tracers that complement FDG by probing biological characteristics of tumors are then discussed.

Min Yao, MD, PhD
Case Western Reserve University
Seidman Cancer Center
University Hospital Case Medical Center
11100 Euclid Avenue
Cleveland, Ohio 44106, USA

Peter F. Faulhaber, MD
Case Western Reserve University
Clinical PET University Hospital Case Medical Center
11100 Euclid Avenue
Cleveland, Ohio 44106, USA

E-mail addresses:
min.yao@uhhospitals.org (M. Yao)
peter.faulhaber@uhhospitals.org (P.F. Faulhaber)

REFERENCES

1. Ha PK, Hdeib A, Goldenberg D, et al. The role of positron emission tomography and computed tomography fusion in the management of early-stage and advanced-stage primary head and neck squamous cell carcinoma. Arch Otolaryngol Head Neck Surg 2006;132(1):12–6.

2. Branstetter BF 4th, Blodgett TM, Zimmer LA, et al. Head and neck malignancy: is PET/CT more accurate than PET or CT alone? Radiology 2005;235(2): 580–6.

PET Clin 7 (2012) xi
http://dx.doi.org/10.1016/j.cpet.2012.08.001
1556-8598/12/$ – see front matter © 2012 Elsevier Inc. All rights reserved.

[^{18}F]Fluorodeoxyglucose-PET/ Computed Tomography, PET, and Magnetic Resonance Imaging
Normal Anatomy, Pitfalls, and Artifacts

Lina Mehta, MD[a,b], Ryan T. Huber, MD[a,c],
Peter F. Faulhaber, MD[b,*]

KEYWORDS

• FDG • Head and neck cancer • Normal variations • PET/CT • PET/MR imaging

KEY POINTS

• 2-[^{18}F]Fluoro-2-deoxy-D-glucose (FDG)-PET/computed tomography (CT) is complementary to anatomic imaging in staging head and neck cancer; a multimodality approach.
• Recognition of normal variations in FDG-PET/CT is critical to accurate interpretation.
• The emerging modality of PET/magnetic resonance imaging shows promise in increasing the accuracy of staging of various malignancies, including head and neck cancer.

INTRODUCTION

This article presents a structured approach to avoiding pitfalls and artifacts in PET/computed tomography (CT) of the head and neck performed with 2-[^{18}F]fluoro-2-deoxy-D-glucose (FDG). A systematic interpretation of an FDG-PET/CT study can take advantage of the TNM (tumor [T], node [N], and metastasis [M]) staging system.[1] Head and neck cancer is an excellent example of the importance FDG-PET/CT in accurate staging. However, FDG-PET/CT can present a particular challenge in the head and neck because the complex anatomy leads to complex physiology, and because the physiology itself can be variable, independently of the anatomy. In addition, prior cancer therapies can lead to altered anatomy and physiology. This article reviews the anatomic and physiologic variations with an emphasis on accurate TNM staging.

PATIENT PREPARATION AND PROTOCOLS

Any procedure in nuclear medicine requires some patient preparation. Patient preparation in oncology is designed to minimize competition of endogenous glucose with FDG and minimize FDG uptake in otherwise normal anatomic areas, such

Disclosure: Dr Faulhaber receives research funding from Philips Medical for an investigator-initiated study of PET/magnetic resonance imaging.
[a] Division of Nuclear Medicine, Department of Radiology, University Case Medical Center, 11100 Euclid Avenue, Cleveland, OH 44106, USA; [b] Case Western Reserve University; [c] Department of Radiology, University Hospitals Case Medical Center
* Corresponding author. Division of Nuclear Medicine, Department of Radiology, University Case Medical Center, 11100 Euclid Avenue, Cleveland, OH 44122.
E-mail address: peter.faulhaber@uhhospitals.org

PET Clin 7 (2012) 345–367
http://dx.doi.org/10.1016/j.cpet.2012.07.001
1556-8598/12/$ – see front matter © 2012 Elsevier Inc. All rights reserved.

as cardiac and skeletal muscle; to minimize these pitfalls, patients are instructed to fast overnight for oncologic PET imaging, but to remain hydrated (no nothing-by-mouth orders). If an overnight fast is not possible, then at least 4 hours is indicated. Blood sugar at the time of FDG administration should be less than 200 mg/dL. In insulin-dependent diabetics, more care is taken to manage blood sugar; management guidelines can be found via the Society of Nuclear Medicine, for example.[2] If blood glucose levels are increased at the time of FDG administration, the administration of insulin to bring blood sugar levels down is not recommended because such an intervention drives glucose, and with it FDG, into skeletal muscles, reducing available FDG uptake in the remainder of the body, including uptake in tumors. Skeletal muscle activation also leads to increased FDG metabolism and patients should, therefore, rest during the radiotracer uptake period. Patients are specifically instructed not to read, because the act of reading can result in increased muscle uptake from flexing the neck and increased ocular muscle activity from eye movement. Of particular importance is instructing the patients not to talk or chew gum during the uptake phase to reduce laryngeal and masticator muscle uptake.

A pattern of neck activity once thought to represent strap muscle and other muscle uptake has been shown by PET/CT to be more commonly caused by brown fat activity with areas of FDG uptake corresponding with areas of adipose tissue. This pattern of uptake was first described by Hany and colleagues[3] in 2002. Many interventions have been described to reduce the amount of brown fat metabolism, and keeping patients warm by advising them to dress warmly, using a warm uptake room, and providing warmed blankets after FDG administration can reduce the brown fat uptake.[4–6]

Protocols for PET/CT head and neck imaging are variable between institutions and also vary depending on indications; variability is caused by factors such as differences in patient positioning, bed positions, and in the use of intravenous (IV) and oral contrast. Protocols also vary according to whether the examination indication is for initial or subsequent therapy evaluation. Our standard protocol for head and neck malignancies is a localized PET/CT acquisition of the head and neck (2 bed positions) with the arms down, followed by PET/CT of the torso with the arms up, from skull base to midthighs. The CT portion for both is non-contrast, low dose. As with any PET/CT, care must be taken between the 2 examinations to avoid motion. In our institution, patients presenting for initial staging have previously received a diagnostic

IV contrast-enhanced scan of the head and neck on a separate CT scanner, and therefore this is not repeated with the PET scan. In certain cases, patients also undergo magnetic resonance (MR) imaging of the head and neck. The additional anatomic images are typically reviewed with PET/CT.

NORMAL ANATOMY AND VARIABLE FDG BIODISTRIBUTION

FDG-PET scans of the head and neck show many areas of mild to moderate uptake that are seen as

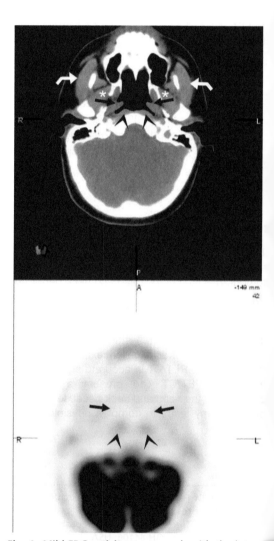

Fig. 1. Mild FDG activity corresponds with the lateral pharyngeal walls (*arrows*) as well as with the longus capitis muscle (*arrowheads*) on the axial CT image reflecting normal physiologic activity. Note the location of the masseter (*curved arrow*) and lateral pterygoid (*asterisk*) muscles.

ormal variants.[7] These areas include the extraoc-
lar eye muscles, salivary glands, and lymphoid
ssue. Muscular activity also is variable and can
e intense with tension, or with recent exercise,
articularly with chewing and phonation. Brown
at activity also can be variable, in location, pat-
ern, and degree of uptake, with FDG metabolism
hat can be at least as intense as that of muscle.
Recognition of these normal variants is critical to
terpretation because tumor staging can be
onfounded by them. Tumor staging varies signif-
cantly with different anatomic regions of the head
and neck; according to the American Joint Committee on Cancer (AJCC) staging system, these
egions are divided into lip and oral cavity,
pharynx, larynx, nasal cavity and paranasal
sinuses, major salivary glands, and thyroid. Al-
hough T staging is the role of anatomic imaging,

variations in FDG uptake can be confounding in
PET/CT. This article therefore reviews the basic
anatomy, physiology, and pitfalls in selected levels
through the head and neck with attention to areas
that confound T staging.

ANATOMIC REGIONS (T STAGING)
Nasopharynx, Oral Cavity, and Oropharynx

Common physiologic pitfalls in the nasopharynx
include lymphoid tissue metabolism and muscular
activity. **Fig. 1** shows an axial PET/CT image at the
nasopharynx with minimal physiologic activity in
the muscles, lateral walls, and sinuses. Lymphoid
tissue can be a cause of false-positives, especially

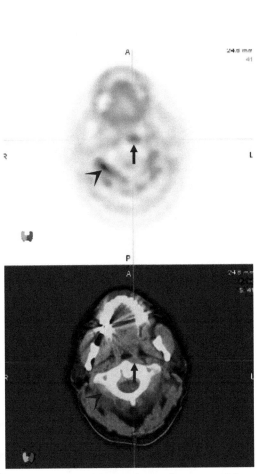

Fig. 2. Longus capitis muscle can be asymmetric, as
shown by the moderate activity (*arrow*). Note asymmetric muscular activity in the posterior neck along
C2 (*arrowhead*).

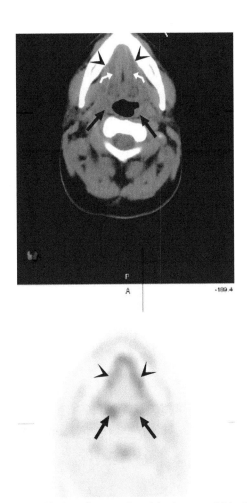

Fig. 3. Mild physiologic FDG activity is seen within the
mylohyoid sling (*arrowheads*) and tonsilar lymphoid
tissue (*arrow*). Mild asymmetry of FDG activity within
the tonsils can be physiologic. No activity is seen in
the genioglossus (*curved arrows*).

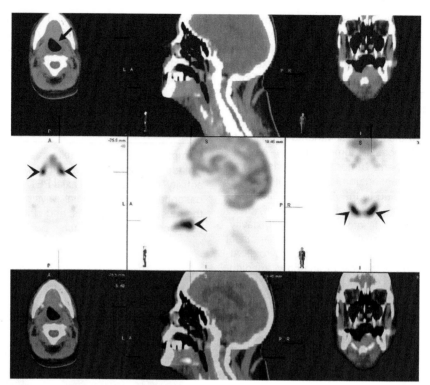

Fig. 4. Increased FDG activity within the mylohyoid sling in a patient with treated tongue base cancer (*arrowheads*) The tongue base is asymmetric without abnormal activity (*arrow*).

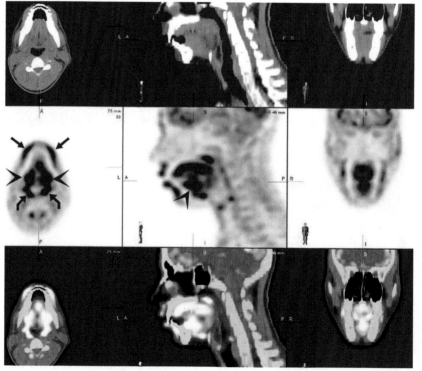

Fig. 5. Example of why insulin should not be administered immediately before FDG injection. The action of insulin drive glucose, and thereby FDG, into cells indiscriminately, resulting in intense muscular uptake. Intense uptake is present throughout the tongue (*arrowheads*), buccal muscles (*arrows*), and pharyngeal walls (*curved arrows*).

younger patients who may show prominent mphoid tissue metabolism, either as a normal ariant or in response to upper respiratory infections. Prevertebral muscular uptake is also common mimic of disorders; symmetric uptake easily discerned as a normal variation but etabolism can be focal or asymmetric, which an be confusing. Correlation with the CT scan nd a recognition of normal patterns of metabom helps exclude disorders. **Fig. 2** shows prominent asymmetric prevertebral muscular activity.

PET/CT images through the oral cavity and opharynx show a wide variation in normal physlogy. **Fig. 3** shows a common pattern of activity, ith mild activity seen in the mylohyoid sling and

tonsils. Activity in the mylohyoid muscle can be prominent, as in **Fig. 4** in a patient with treated tongue base cancer. A pattern of muscular uptake is shown in **Fig. 5** in a patient who received insulin before PET imaging. Localizing disorders in such a setting would be limited.

Larynx

Laryngeal uptake can be variable but is usually symmetric, reflecting the paired laryngeal muscles.[8] As mentioned earlier, patients should be encouraged to refrain from phonation after tracer injection to decrease the metabolism in the vocal cord muscles. **Fig. 6** shows a typical pattern of activity at the laryngeal level. Asymmetric activity can be seen in the setting of vocal cord paralysis with the normal side showing increased activity compared with the abnormal side. Abnormal FDG uptake in the vocal cords can be increased after injection laryngoplasty, often with Teflon or other augmentation materials such as collagen derivatives. Such injections can cause a granulomatous reaction leading to a potentially false-positive PET.[9] Knowledge of

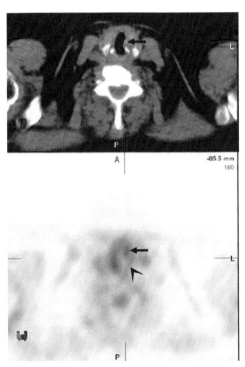

Fig. 7. Appearance of the left vocal cord by CT as a result of treatment of vocal cord paralysis with injection laryngoplasty (*arrow*). However, the associated FDG activity is decreased at the cricoarytenoid (*arrowhead*).

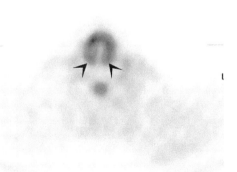

ig. 6. Symmetric physiologic FDG activity within the ocal cords; an upside-down horseshoe shape with he bases at the cricoarytenoid muscles (*arrowheads*).

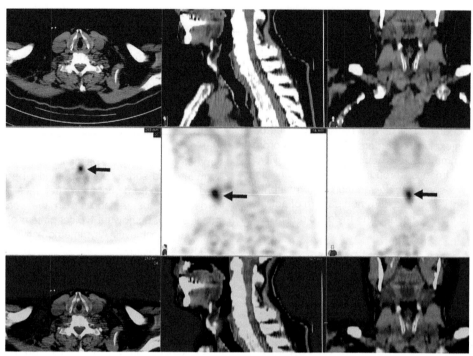

Fig. 8. Focal FDG activity at the anterior commissure of the vocal cords indicates a true laryngeal neoplasm (*arrow*). The corresponding CT images are misleadingly unremarkable.

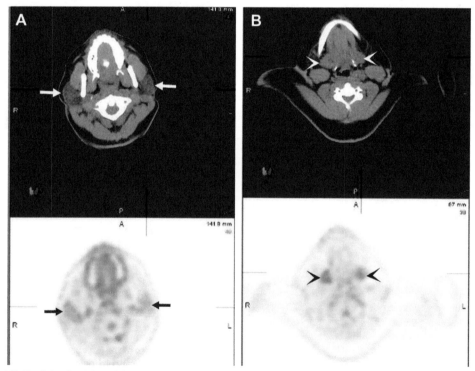

Fig. 9. (*A*) Physiologic FDG activity is seen corresponding with the bilateral parotid glands (*arrows*). (*B*) Physiologic FDG activity is seen corresponding with the bilateral submandibular glands (*arrowheads*).

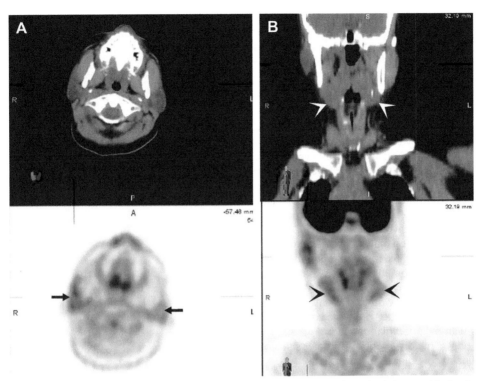

Fig. 10. (A) Increased FDG activity is seen in the right parotid gland more than the left parotid gland on axial images (arrows). (B) Coronal images again show increased FDG activity in the right parotid gland, but now also show increased activity in the bilateral submandibular glands (arrowheads). The pattern of activity, given that this patient received I-131 therapy for thyroid cancer, helps distinguish this appearance of radiation sialadenitis from other pathologic processes.

such previous surgical interventions is critical for accurate interpretations. A patient after silicone injection to the left vocal cord is shown in **Fig. 7.** **Fig. 8** shows a patient with a small laryngeal primary at the anterior commissure without a corresponding anatomic abnormality.

Salivary Glands

Activity in the salivary glands is variable and can be asymmetric. The highest activity is typically seen in the parotid and submandibular glands. Sublingual activity typically is mild and can be difficult to distinguish from the mylohyoid sling. Salivary activity can be asymmetric. Normal parotid and submandibular glands are shown in **Fig. 9.** A patient with increased and asymmetric salivary activity in the clinical setting of thyroidectomy and I-131 radioiodine therapy is shown in **Fig. 10.** The increased activity is thought to reflect sialadenitis from the radioiodine therapy. Focal uptake is often associated with neoplasm, as shown in a study of

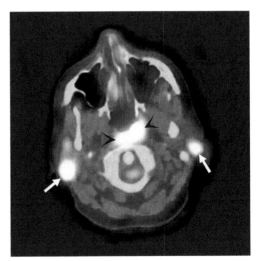

Fig. 11. Focal FDG uptake in the bilateral parotid glands (arrows) in a patient with pancreatic cancer. Note that the activity does not encompass the entirety of the glands and represents Warthin tumors, which are often bilateral. Activity is also present in the posterior nasopharynx, which is inflammatory (arrowheads).

parotid uptake on PET by Basu and colleagues[10] in a study of focally increased parotid uptake on FDG-PET. A patient with bilateral focal parotid uptake is shown in **Fig. 11**. These foci were shown to be Warthin tumors, which can be bilateral.

Thyroid Gland

Thyroid activity is variable and should be interpreted with caution when seen in routine oncologic PET. In general, diffuse and irregular thyroid activity usually has a benign cause, commonly thyroiditis. Focal activity is more frequently caused by malignancy. Kwak and colleagues[11] studied 87 patients with focal thyroid uptake on FDG-PET, and found 48.3% to be malignant; the percentage of malignancy was 75.5% when correlated with suspicious findings on ultrasound. A patient with an FDG-avid left thyroid nodule is presented in **Fig. 12**. This nodule was malignant at biopsy. Thyroid uptake can be dramatic at times in patients with enlarged glands, as in **Fig. 13**. This patient has a history of both sarcoidosis (note mediastinal focal uptake) and thyroiditis.

NODAL REGIONS (N STAGING) AND VARIABLE FDG DISTRIBUTION

The recent seventh edition of the AJCC cancer staging manual made no changes to the nodal staging of head and neck malignancies.[1] The lack of N-stage changes likely reflects the continued importance of nodal status for patient prognosis. Prognosis is worse with an increased number of nodes, nodes in the lower neck, and extracapsular spread. FDG-PET alone was documented by various studies to be more sensitive than CT or MR imaging for nodal assessment. For example, Wong and colleagues[12] showed a sensitivity of 67% and a specificity of 100% compared with sensitivity and specificity of CT/MR imaging at 67% and 25%. Many studies subsequently documented the superiority of PET/CT for staging head and neck malignancies relative to PET or CT by themselves, such as the study by Barnstetter and colleagues.[13] Therefore it is important to recognize the nodal levels and variations in FDG uptake to avoid misdiagnosis.

The regional lymph nodes in the head and neck are typically divided into subsets and grouped into 7 levels (also see the article elsewhere in this issue):

1. Submental and submandibular
2. Upper jugular
3. Middle jugular
4. Lower jugular
5. Posterior triangle
6. Prelaryngeal, pretracheal, paratracheal
7. Upper mediastinal

Lymph node localization into these levels is typically done at the time of diagnostic CT with IV

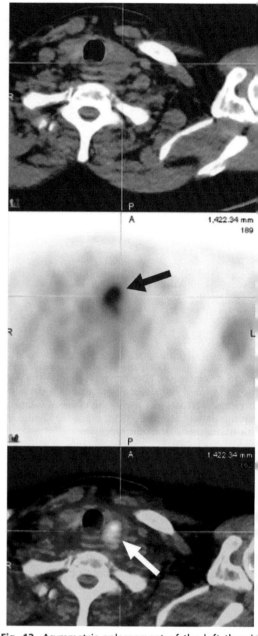

Fig. 12. Asymmetric enlargement of the left thyroid gland. Note the focal FDG activity (*arrow*): biopsy of this region yielded thyroid malignancy.

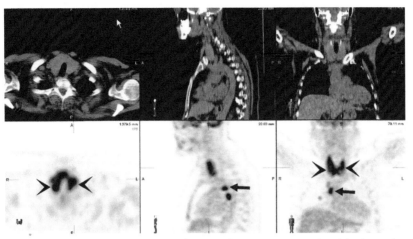

g. 13. Diffuse enlargement of the thyroid gland with intense heterogeneous FDG activity (*arrowheads*), in this case lated to Hashimoto thyroiditis. Note that this patient also has sarcoidosis, with focal mediastinal uptake (*arrow*).

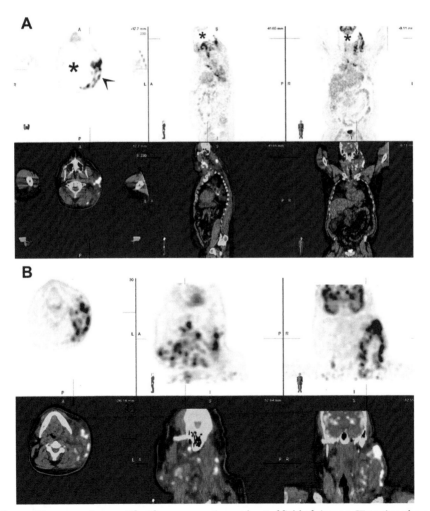

ig. 14. (*A*) Torso with arms up shows artifact from arm motion and out of field of view on CT causing photopenic defect cross right neck (*asterisk*). The patient has extensive left neck adenopathy (*arrowhead*). (*B*) Images of the head and neck vith arms down show no artifact. Extensive lymphadenopathy in the left neck is more clearly seen.

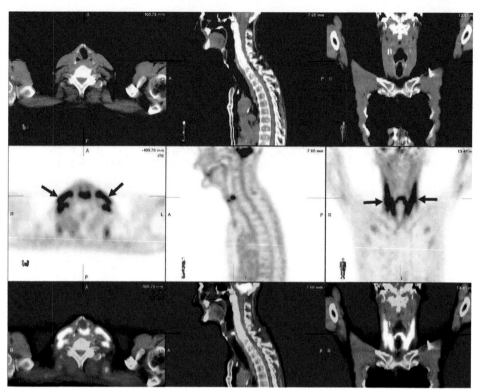

Fig. 15. Patient with prominent FDG activity in the sternocleidomastoid (*arrows*). This activity can mask subtle lymph nodal activity, especially in patients such as this with scarce fat planes.

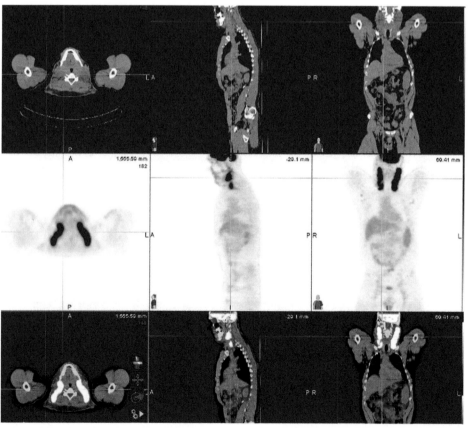

Fig. 16. Symmetric bilateral cervical FDG activity, in this case representing enlarged confluent cervical lymph nodes. Note the subtle nodularity that differentiates this from muscular activity.

ontrast enhancement. PET/CT can be less accu-
ate than IV contrast–enhanced CT in nodal local-
ation if the CT is low dose noncontrast.
evertheless, PET/CT interpretations should
clude regional localization of lymph node activity
s much as possible. Pitfalls in nodal staging can
ccur secondary to technical errors, brown fat
ctivity, and variable muscle activation. Errors of
lignment between the CT and PET images result
 incorrect attenuation. This error is more
ommon with PET images obtained with the
rms elevated, as in **Fig. 14A**. The abnormality is
ot seen with the arms down in head and neck
nages (see **Fig. 14B**). Extensive neck muscle
ptake can be confounding in lymph node assess-
ent, especially in a patient with little body fat, as
 Fig. 15. In contrast, **Fig. 16** shows a similar
attern of V-shaped anterior cervical activity that
epresents extensive symmetric nodes. Some-
mes both brown fat and lymph node activity
ccur at the same time in a patient. In such

a setting, close inspection of the CT helps separate lymph node from brown fat, as in **Fig. 17**;
the degree of uptake cannot be used to distinguish
between a malignant node and brown fat. Focal
activity from brown fat can also extend into the
mediastinum along the great vessels. When the
extension occurs in the context of a typical pattern
in the neck and torso, clinicians can be confident
of the correct diagnosis. However, focal mediastinal uptake can occur in isolation, as shown in
Fig. 18. Close inspection of the CT shows the
activity adjacent to the great vessels of the aortic
arch.

Muscular uptake can be focal, mimicking lymph
node activity, or diffuse, suggesting extensive
tumor invasion. Focal uptake in 1 plane, such as
axial, can look focal, but appear linear in another
plane. A linear pattern is more typical of a benign
finding such as muscle. **Fig. 19** shows a patient
with extensive muscular uptake secondary to grimacing in pain during the uptake phase. The

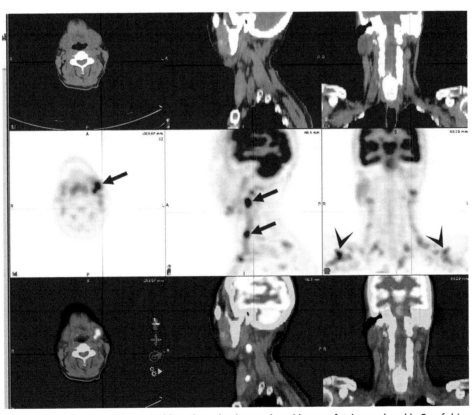

Fig. 17. FDG activity seen in both cervical lymph nodes (*arrows*) and brown fat (*arrowheads*). Careful inspection
of the CT images reveals FDG-avid foci corresponding with regions of fat attenuation as potentially confounding
brown fat.

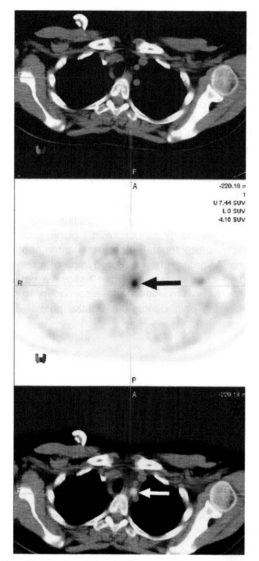

Fig. 18. Focal uptake in the superior mediastinum suggesting an FDG-avid lymph node corresponds with fat between the great vessel origins (*arrow*) and is identified as brown fat.

abnormal lymph node is less intense than the muscle.

Metastatic Disease

Distant metastatic disease is uncommon in squamous cell carcinoma of the head and neck at presentation. The cancer tends to remain localized to the primary site and regional nodes. At the time of diagnosis, regional lymph node involvement is present in 43% and metastatic disease in 10% of

patients.[14] Risk factors for the development of metastatic disease were retrospectively evaluated in 1972 patients by Garavello and colleagues. These risk factors were younger age (<45 years), hypopharyngeal location, advanced T or N stage, high histologic grade, and locoregional recurrence. The rate of distant metastases was 9.2%. The most common metastatic site was lung (55.8%). Patients are also at risk of second primary tumors. A large cancer registry study showed that the most common second primary was lung cancer, with a 20-year cumulative risk of 13%.[16,1] **Fig. 20.** shows a patient with a new lung nodule after diagnosis of head and neck cancer. With the current generation of PET/CT instruments, small lesions can be detected, as in **Fig. 21.** I lesions less than 1 cm, the FDG uptake activity of the lesion is reduced by the volume-averaging effect and thus appears mild. Lymph node activity in the hila and mediastinum can be seen as well, and is often inflammatory, especially in regions with a high prevalence of histoplasmosis, as in **Fig. 22.** Such an uptake pattern at staging of head and neck cancer is unlikely to be metastatic.

MULTIMODALITY IMAGING
PET/CT and MR Imaging

Combining the strengths of anatomic and physiologic imaging can offer more accurate staging. Tumor staging is best accomplished with anatomic imaging, typically MR imaging, whereas nodal and metastatic evaluation is best accomplished with PET (primarily PET/CT). These modalities are combined for a complete assessment. PET images can be fused with MR images using software to take advantage of both modalities. Such a fusion can be done with a high degree of accuracy if attention is paid to patient positioning. There have been several studies evaluating fused PET and MR images compared with PET/CT, CT and MR imaging by themselves. For example, a study by Huang and colleagues on advanced buccal squamous cell carcinoma showed that PET and MR imaging had the highest sensitivity and specificity for assessment of focal invasion and tumor size delineation. PET and MR imaging depict tumor location and focal invasion better than PET/CT, especially in areas of complex anatomy such as the nasopharynx. There is only 1 PET image set of the head and neck to select for fusion, but many sequence choices from the MR imaging study. The MR imaging protocol of the head and neck for staging at our institution includes T2 axial fat saturation (FS), T1 axial, T1 sagittal, and T1 coronal and axial with contrast

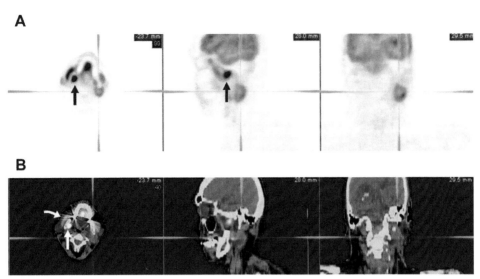

Fig. 19. (A) Intense focal FDG activity posterior to the right maxilla (*arrow*), and less impressive heterogeneous activity in the left upper cervical region (*green crosshairs*). (B) Overlay with CT imaging shows the intense focal activity previously seen within the right medial pterygoid muscle (*arrow*), caused by patient grimacing. Activity is also seen in the right masseter muscle (*curved arrow*). The less intense heterogeneous FDG activity acquires new significance when seen in a region of upper cervical lymphadenopathy (*green crosshair*).

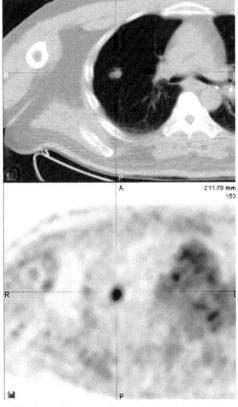

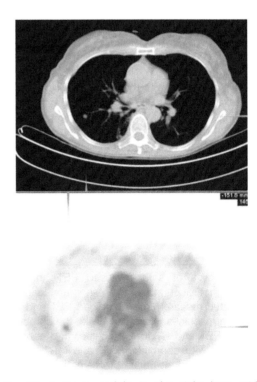

Fig. 20. Axial CT image through the chest and corresponding PET image showing new hypermetabolic right upper lobe pulmonary nodule in a patient diagnosed with head and neck cancer.

Fig. 21. A 5-mm nodule in the right lung with moderate uptake in a patient with history of a parotid malignancy was a metastatic lesion at resection. Current PET/CT technology allows detection of smaller hypermetabolic pulmonary nodules, potentially in the subcentimeter/millimeter range.

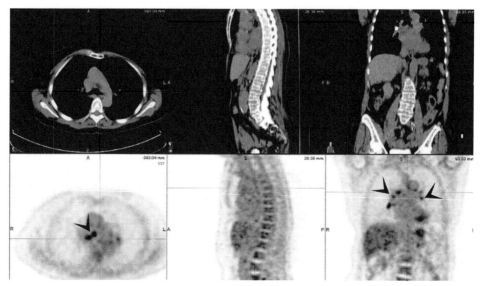

Fig. 22. Prominent mediastinal and hilar nodes (*arrowheads*) with increased FDG activity in a Midwestern patient with histoplasmosis suggests the possibility of disseminated metastatic disease. Although not fully included, a lack of significant nodal activity in the neck makes metastases from head and neck cancer unlikely, particularly at initial staging.

We typically start with the T2 axial FS for fusion. For example, **Fig. 23** compares PET and MR imaging with PET/CT in a patient with a new diagnosis of nasopharyngeal carcinoma. The MR images display the tumor in the left nasopharynx and also show extension along the vidian nerve. The low-dose CT primarily shows abnormal soft tissue and anatomic distortion. **Fig. 24** shows a patient after completion of chemoradiation with resolution of the primary tumor and lymph node.

PET/MR Imaging

The success of software-fused PET and MR imaging for accurate staging in many cancers stimulated research into combined PET and MR imaging machines. However, unlike the combination of PET and CT in 1 machine, the technical problems with combining PET and MR imaging are greater. Among these problems is the effect of the magnetic field on the PET instrument and the need to calculate photon attenuation data from MR imaging data. With PET/CT, the distribution of photon attenuation coefficients (attenuation map) is derived from the distribution of Hounsfield units on CT scaled to 511-keV attenuation units.[18]

Calculating an attenuation map from an MR image creates a different problem because MR imaging does not measure tissue density but rather proton density and magnetization relaxation. In addition, MR imaging does not easily distinguish cortical bone from air. One solution to the problem involves segmenting tissue into specific types for attenuation correction. For example, Zaidi and colleagues[19] showed the possibility of creating an attenuation map from a T1-weighted MR image. They created an automated method that defines attenuation for soft tissue, lungs, and air. Newer methods attempt to segment tissue into bone, soft tissue, lung, and air using ultrashort echo time MR images. These methods create MR attenuation-corrected PET images that compare with CT attenuation-corrected PET images with clinically acceptable errors.

The problem of the magnetic field's impact on the PET instrument has 2 current solutions. One is physical separation of the 2 instruments and shielding of the PET. The other is a PET insert inside the MR imaging magnet. The first method is effectively sequential, much like PET/CT, whereas the second is simultaneous. A study by Schlemmer and colleagues[20] showed the feasibility of

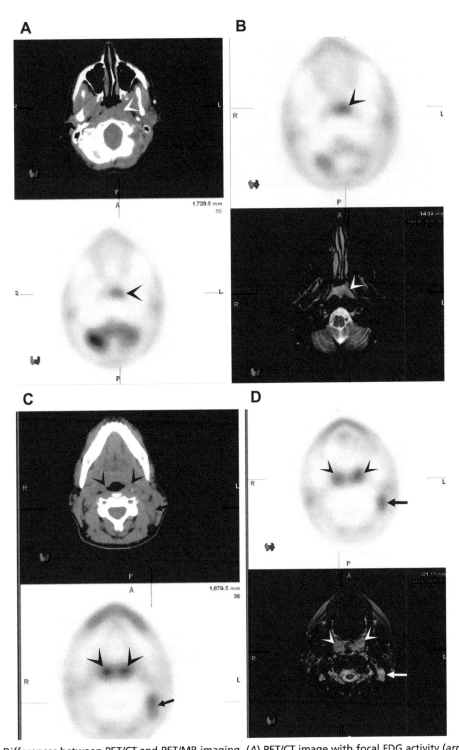

Fig. 23. Differences between PET/CT and PET/MR imaging. (*A*) PET/CT image with focal FDG activity (*arrowhead*) shows the location of a left nasopharyngeal carcinoma, in a region of increased soft tissue and architectural distortion. (*B*) PET and MR imaging show that the focal uptake corresponds with abnormal signal in the left posterior nasopharynx (*arrowhead*); the images are better defined than those from CT. (*C*) PET/CT image shows a left malignant node (*arrow*) and physiologic uptake in the pharyngeal tonsils (*arrowheads*). (*D*) PET and MR imaging images show the left malignant node (*arrow*) and physiologic uptake in the tonsils (*arrowhead*). The tissue signal of the tonsils is better defined on MR imaging than on CT.

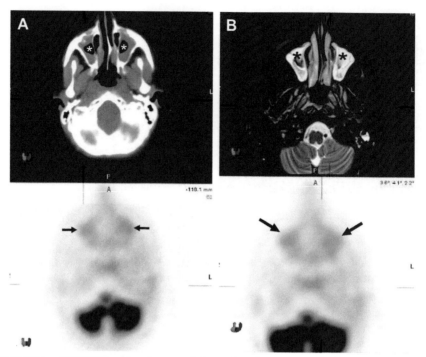

Fig. 24. (*A, B*) PET/CT and PET/MR imaging images of the patient from **Fig. 23** showing resolution of tumor after chemotherapy. Mild uptake is present in the maxillary sinuses (*arrows*) corresponding with soft tissue thickening increased signal on CT and MR imaging (*asterisk*).

a simultaneous PET/MR imaging instrument with a PET ring mounted inside a 3-T MR imaging machine. The performance of a sequential PET/MR imaging system from Philips was documented in a study by Zaidi and colleagues that showed that the PET subsystem was comparable with a similar PET subsystem in PET/CT. The PET and MR imaging instruments are separated by 3 m with a common scanning bed between.

At our institution, we have begun experimental studies on a sequential PET/MR imaging instrument (Philips Ingenuity TF PET/MR). The instrument combines a time of flight (TF) PET system combined with 3-T MR imaging. We are using a fast T1-weighted MR sequence of the torso (matching PET/CT) to generate a segmented attenuation map of air, lung, and soft tissue to correct the PET images. **Fig. 25** shows PET/MR imaging of the torso for a patient with treated tongue cancer. The patient has had a right partial glossectomy and pharyngectomy with mandibular reconstruction. The images were acquired approximately 50 minutes after clinical PET/CT. The MR imaging sequence used for

the attenuation map lacks the fine anatomic detail of the CT portion of PET/CT. Additional MR sequences, as in diagnostic MR imaging, are needed for anatomic detail. **Fig. 26** shows additional MR sequences of the head and neck coregistered with the PET images. The images show significant tongue uptake with no corresponding abnormality on either CT or MR imaging. Magnetic susceptibility artifact is noted as well from a right mandibular reconstruction. An additional patient with treated tongue cancer with left glossectomy and flap reconstruction showed significant tongue uptake in PET/CT, as shown in **Fig. 27**. Subsequent PET/MR imaging shows a similar pattern. There were no abnormal findings on physical examination.

Research is continuing to develop attenuation maps from MR imaging data. A recent article by Berker and colleagues[21] shows the feasibility of classification-based MR imaging attenuation correction accounting for 4 different tissue classes (cortical bone, air, adipose tissue, and soft tissue) by combining the ultrashort echo time triple-echo MR imaging sequence with

A

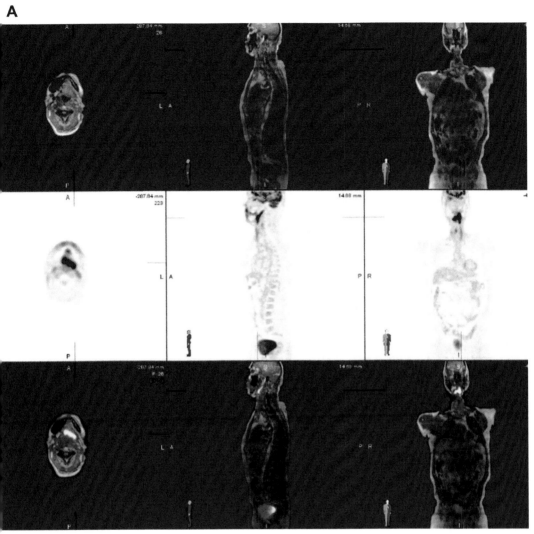

Fig. 25. PET/MR imaging (*A*) and PET/CT (*B*) of the torso with treated tongue cancer, following right partial glossec-tomy, pharyngectomy, and mandibular reconstruction. Note that the T1 MR attenuation map lacks the anatomic detail to outline these extensive postoperative changes; additional diagnostic MR sequences are required.

dedicated postprocessing, exploiting the benefits of ultrashort echo time acquisition as well as Dixon. A clinical study by Drzezga and colleagues[22] summarized experience with integrated PET/MR to PET/CT in oncology. They found that Dixon MR imaging sequences acquired for attenuation correction allowed good anatomic allocation of PET findings. A future PET/MR imaging protocol

in head and neck cancer might consist of tracer administration followed by an attenuation scan and dedicated MR imaging of the head and neck during the uptake phase, with subsequent PET scan of the head and neck. Dixon MR imaging sequences of the torso might be followed by PET of the torso for evaluation of metastatic disease.

B

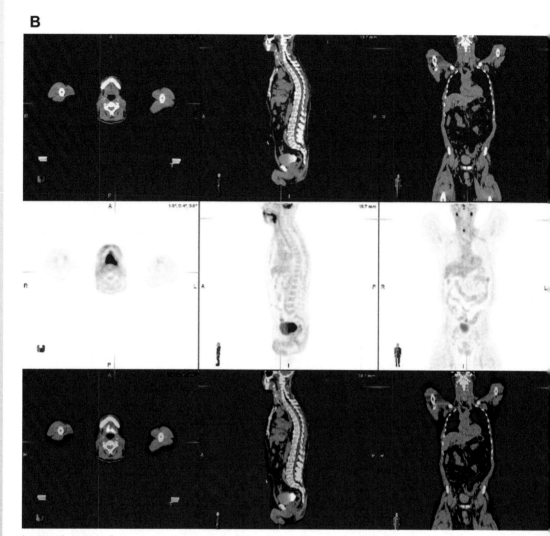

Fig. 25. (*continued*)

A

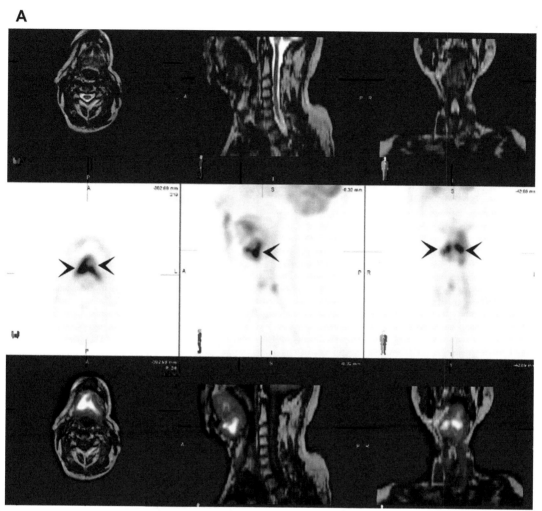

Fig. 26. The same patient as in Fig. 25, focusing on the head and neck. (A) Additional T2 axial MR imaging sequence registered to PET showing prominent FDG activity in the tongue (*arrowheads*), without corresponding abnormalities on MR imaging. (B) PET/MR imaging T1 sequence and PET/CT images of the head and neck showing magnetic susceptibility artifact (*arrow*) from mandibular reconstruction (*arrowhead*) and intense uptake in tongue. (C) PET/MR imaging T1 sequence shows absent left vocal cord activity (*arrows*). MR imaging shows bulging left vocal cord (*arrowhead*). (D) PET/CT showing absent left vocal cord activity.

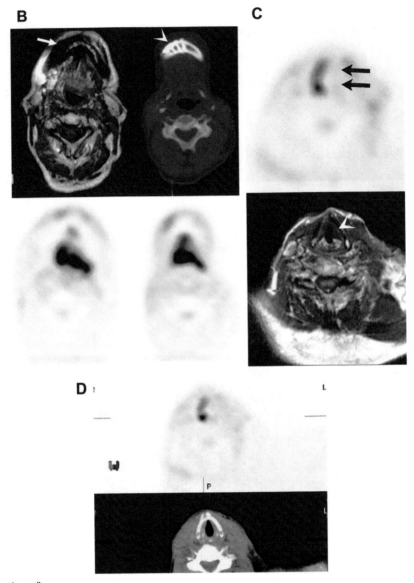

Fig. 26. (continued)

A

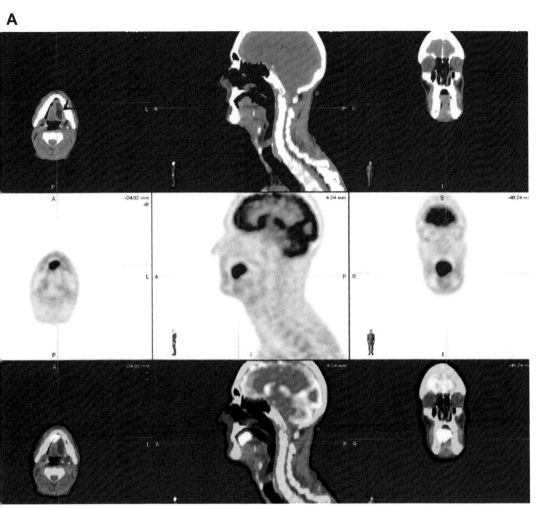

Fig. 27. PET/CT (*A*) and PET/MR imaging (*B*) of a patient following left glossectomy and flap reconstruction. Prominent FDG activity is seen within the anterior tongue despite no abnormalities on imaging or physical examination. The left tongue reconstruction is seen as fat on both the CT and MR imaging sequences (*arrowhead*). The MR images are from the T1 axial attenuation correction map of the torso.

B

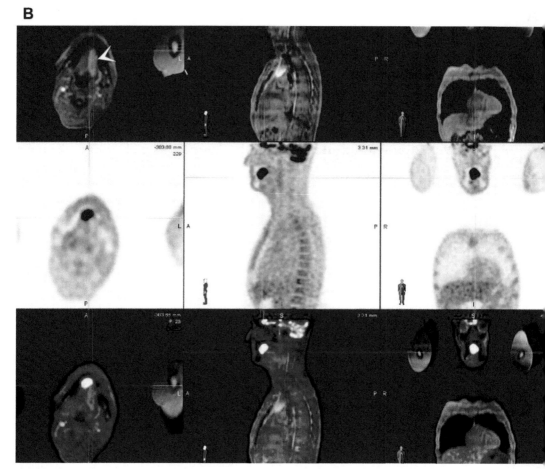

Fig. 27. (*continued*)

SUMMARY

Each anatomic region of the head and neck has physiologic variations that can mimic a primary tumor or lymph node. Many of these variations can be recognized as reflecting benign lymphoid, salivary, brown fat, and muscular activity. A few artifacts are related to CT attenuation. A knowledge of tumor types and patterns of lymph node and metastatic spread helps categorize patterns as benign or malignant.

The anatomic reference of CT helps solve many pitfalls. A recently introduced instrument, PET/MR imaging, will face new pitfalls as its role in oncology is developed.

ACKNOWLEDGMENTS

Figure Editor: Joseph P. Molter, Manager of Medical Photography, Case Center for Imaging Research.

REFERENCES

1. Rice TW, Blackstone EH, Rusch VW. 7th edition of the AJCC Cancer Staging Manual: esophagus and esophagogastric junction. Ann Surg Oncol 2010; 17(7):1721–4.
2. Fletcher JW, et al. Recommendations on the use of 18F-FDG PET in oncology. J Nucl Med 2008;49(3): 480–508.
3. Hany TF, et al. Brown adipose tissue: a factor to consider in symmetrical tracer uptake in the neck and upper chest region. Eur J Nucl Med Mol Imaging 2002;29(10):1393–8.
4. Gelfand MJ, et al. Pre-medication to block [(18)F] FDG uptake in the brown adipose tissue of pediatric and adolescent patients. Pediatr Radiol 2005; 35(10):984–90.
5. Soderlund V, Larsson SA, Jacobsson H. Reduction of FDG uptake in brown adipose tissue in clinical patients by a single dose of propranolol. Eur J Nucl Med Mol Imaging 2007;34(7):1018–22.

6. Tatsumi M, et al. Intense (18)F-FDG uptake in brown fat can be reduced pharmacologically. J Nucl Med 2004;45(7):1189–93.

7. Jabour BA, et al. Extracranial head and neck: PET imaging with 2-[F-18]fluoro-2-deoxy-D-glucose and MR imaging correlation. Radiology 1993;186(1):27–35.

8. Kostakoglu L, et al. Speech-related visualization of laryngeal muscles with fluorine-18-FDG. J Nucl Med 1996;37(11):1771–3.

9. Yeretsian RA, et al. Teflon-induced granuloma: a false-positive finding with PET resolved with combined PET and CT. AJNR Am J Neuroradiol 2003;24(6):1164–6.

10. Basu S, Houseni M, Alavi A. Significance of incidental fluorodeoxyglucose uptake in the parotid glands and its impact on patient management. Nucl Med Commun 2008;29(4):367–73.

11. Kwak JY, et al. Thyroid incidentalomas identified by 18F-FDG PET: sonographic correlation. AJR Am J Roentgenol 2008;191(2):598–603.

12. Wong WL, et al. A prospective study of PET-FDG imaging for the assessment of head and neck squamous cell carcinoma. Clin Otolaryngol Allied Sci 1997;22(3):209–14.

13. Branstetter BF, et al. Head and neck malignancy: is PET/CT more accurate than PET or CT alone? Radiology 2005;235(2):580–6.

14. Ridge JA, GB, Lango MN, et al. Head and neck tumors. In: Haller DG, Wagman LD, Camphausen KA, et al, editor. Cancer management. 14th edition; 2011, Oncology.

15. Garavello W, et al. Risk factors for distant metastases in head and neck squamous cell carcinoma. Arch Otolaryngol Head Neck Surg 2006;132(7):762–6.

16. Chuang SC, et al. Risk of second primary cancer among patients with head and neck cancers: a pooled analysis of 13 cancer registries. Int J Cancer 2008;123(10):2390–6.

17. Chuang SC, et al. Risk of second primary cancer among esophageal cancer patients: a pooled analysis of 13 cancer registries. Cancer Epidemiol Biomarkers Prev 2008;17(6):1543–9.

18. Beyer T, et al. A combined PET/CT scanner for clinical oncology. J Nucl Med 2000;41(8):1369–79.

19. Keereman V, et al. MRI-based attenuation correction for PET/MRI using ultrashort echo time sequences. J Nucl Med 2010;51(5):812–8.

20. Schlemmer HP, et al. Simultaneous MR/PET imaging of the human brain: feasibility study. Radiology 2008;248(3):1028–35.

21. Berker Y, et al. MRI-based attenuation correction for hybrid PET/MRI systems: a 4-class tissue segmentation technique using a combined ultrashort-echo-time/Dixon MRI sequence. J Nucl Med 2012;53(5):796–804.

22. Drzezga A, et al. First clinical experience with integrated whole-body PET/MR: comparison to PET/CT in patients with oncologic diagnoses. J Nucl Med 2012;53(6):845–55.

FDG-PET/CT Initial and Subsequent Therapy Evaluation

Progressing to PET/MR Imaging

Camila Mosci, MD, Guido A. Davidzon, MD, Andrew Quon, MD*

KEYWORDS

- Head and neck cancer • ^{18}F-FDG • PET/CT • PET/MR imaging

KEY POINTS

- ^{18}F-2-fluoro-2-deoxy-D-glucose (FDG) PET/computed tomography (CT) has become a widely used imaging modality for a variety of malignancies and is increasingly becoming a standard part of the management of head and neck cancer (HNC).
- The benefits of ^{18}F-FDG PET/CT include initial staging, monitoring of the response of therapy, and surveillance.
- PET/MR imaging is a new promising imaging modality that combines the excellent anatomic resolution and high soft-tissue contrast of MR imaging with the high sensitive evaluation of metabolism achieved with PET.

INTRODUCTION

Worldwide, head and neck cancer (HNC) has an estimated incidence of 965,728 and estimated mortality of 681,346, annually.[1] The estimated incidence and mortality for this type of tumor in the United States is 40,250 and 7850, respectively.[2] Nasopharyngeal cancer has an incidence as high as 25 per 100,000 in Southern China, and in India, head and neck squamous cell carcinoma (HNSCC) accounts for 25% of all male carcinomas and 10% of all female carcinomas.[3,4] More than two-thirds of patients with HNSCC initially present with advanced stage (American Joint Committee on Cancer Stage III–IVB). Of these patients, traditionally, less than one-half will have local disease control with nonoperative therapy and even fewer (between 20% and 40%) will survive 3 years after their diagnosis.[5]

Therapy often requires extensive multidisciplinary collaboration among specialists in head and neck surgery, radiation oncology, medical oncology, prosthodontics, and speech therapy. Diagnostic imaging plays an important role in accurate staging, restaging, and treatment monitoring and is essential both in planning adequate treatment and in minimizing treatment-related toxicity and functional impairment. Magnetic resonance imaging (MR imaging) and computed tomography (CT) remain the primary imaging modalities for the assessment of HNSCC. However, these modalities have been proved ineffective in some cases as the early detection of residual or recurrent foci.[6,7] The contrast among muscular, connective, and cancerous tissue is sometimes difficult to assess. Tumors of the larynx are particularly difficult to interpret, and there are known interobserver differences when estimating the tumor volume. Metastatic

Division of Nuclear Medicine, Stanford University Medical Center, 300 Pasteur Drive, Room H-0250, Stanford, CA 94305, USA
* Corresponding author.
E-mail address: aquon@stanford.edu

PET Clin 7 (2012) 369–380
http://dx.doi.org/10.1016/j.cpet.2012.06.002
1556-8598/12/$ – see front matter © 2012 Published by Elsevier Inc.

lymph nodes are usually assessed depending on their size (eg, 8–15 mm) and shape (eg, round), and there is the risk of missing small tumors. Hence, PET/CT and PET/MR imaging have emerged as adjunct imaging modalities.

The use of FDG PET/CT for the evaluation of HNC has been most widely assessed for HNSCC, although it has also been studied for other malignancies such as those of salivary gland and thyroid origin. PET/CT rarely adds additional useful information regarding the initial T-stage of the primary tumor because the combination of clinical mucosal evaluation and MR imaging or CT better evaluates local soft tissue and bony anatomy. PET/CT can be helpful, however, in several clinical scenarios: (1) delineation of extent of regional nodal involvement, (2) detection of distant metastases, (3) identification of an unknown primary, (4) detection of the occasional synchronous primary, (5) monitoring treatment response, and (6) long-term surveillance for recurrence and metastases.

INITIAL STAGING OF SQUAMOUS CELL CARCINOMA OF THE HEAD AND NECK

Accurate delineation of the primary tumor and the extent of regional nodal metastases are critical for the staging of the tumor, for determination of the optimal initial therapeutic approach (extent of surgery and targets for radiation therapy), and for survival rate. For example, the presence of lymph node metastases is one of the most important prognostic factors, and patients with confirmed nodal involvement have a considerable reduction of their 5-year survival rate.[8]

Although numerous reports on initial staging have shown that PET is at least as sensitive as MR imaging or CT in detecting the primary tumor,[9–11] PET and PET/CT (without contrast) lack the anatomic definition that MR imaging and contrast-enhanced multislice CT can provide. Therefore, there is little role for PET in defining the T-stage of the primary tumor. One exception is the utility of FDG PET in identifying the primary tumor site in patients who present with metastatic HNSCC in the cervical nodes from a clinically undetectable or unknown primary tumor, which is discussed further in the next section.

Conventional imaging such as CT and MR imaging are the initial imaging studies for staging head and neck tumors. When compared with PET/CT without contrast, MR imaging is capable of more accurately delineating the extent of tumor and evaluating perineural involvement and intracranial extension of disease and is nearly comparable in accuracy in detecting regional nodal metastases.[12,13] A contrast-enhanced CT is mostly used in cases of laryngeal cancer. However, the merit of MR imaging over contrast-enhanced CT is still deeply debated between institutions, and a combined PET/CT performed with intravenous contrast may be a reasonably accurate alternative for delineating the extent of disease at initial presentation.[?]

For evaluating metastatic cervical lymph nodes, previous studies have shown that FDG PET/CT is at least comparable or superior to conventional imaging in detecting regional nodal metastases in initial staging (**Fig. 1**).[15–18] However, its role in the evaluation of normal size lymph nodes is controversial, and its major advantage may lie in

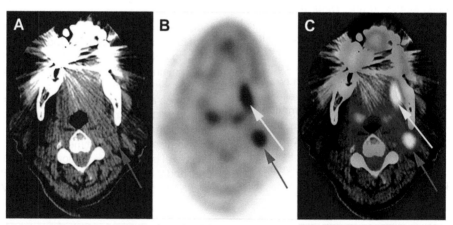

Fig. 1. Detection of malignant lymph node at initial staging. An 80-year-old woman with 4 months history of swallowing difficulty and white patches on left tongue for which biopsy revealed moderate differentiated squamous cell carcinoma. (*A*) Low-resolution CT, (*B*) FDG PET, and (*C*) fusion PET/CT showed the primary tumor on the left lateral tongue (*yellow arrows*) as well as an enlarged hypermetabolic left level II lymph node suspicious for metastasis (*blue arrows*). She had left partial glossectomy and left modified radical neck dissection that confirmed primary tumor and metastatic carcinoma.

he differentiation of normal from abnormal FDG ccumulations. It is important to consider that he presence of small lesions, low tumor metabolic ctivity, and hyperglycemia may yield false-egative FDG-PET results.[19] A review by Schoder nd Yeung[13] reported an average sensitivity of 7% to 90% and specificity of 80% to 93% for DG PET/CT as compared with a sensitivity of 1% to 97% and specificity of 21% to 100% for he combination of MR imaging and CT. Another tudy suggested that MR imaging may be slightly nore sensitive than PET for identifying regional nodal metastases (93% for MR imaging vs 85% or PET).[20] Specificity was comparable between he 2 imaging modalities (95% for MR imaging vs 8% for PET). However, this study used a nonhy-brid PET scanner without PET/CT fusion; inte-grated PET/CT scanning may be as good as or better than both MR imaging and PET used alone.

FDG PET/CT does not perform as well for nodal staging as it does for assessment of distant meta-static diseases. In patients who are clinically stage N0 after initial evaluation (no evidence of nodal nvolvement by physical examination and anatomic imaging), 2 small studies using sentinel ymph node biopsy as a gold standard showed hat PET failed to detect malignant lymph nodes n 8 out of 9 patients (from both studies collec-ively).[21,22] A larger prospective study report of 31 stage N0 patients showed that FDG PET/CT ailed to detect minimally involved ($\leq$3 mm) lymph nodes in 3 patients and had false-positive findings n 4.[23] The most likely cause of false-negative esults is the limited spatial resolution of PET and ts poor performance in detecting lesions less han 5 mm. Therefore, a selective neck dissection or a sentinel lymph node biopsy is more definitive.

Even in patients with clinically N0 disease, a PET/CT scan at the time of initial staging may still serve as a useful baseline examination for subsequent follow-up after therapy (see later discussion) and should be included as an optional measure. It is particularly useful to have a baseline PET/CT scan to help differentiate incidental physiologic FDG-avid foci from malignant foci on subsequent post-treatment scans. Normal variant FDG uptake is seen in a variety of locations, including the pharyn-geal muscles, salivary glands, and lymphoid tissue and may pose a significant interpretive challenge when comparison images are not available.

HNC has a high propensity for developing distant metastases and second primary cancers, ranging rom 6.1% to 16% and for becoming the leading cause of treatment failure and death in these patients.[24] FDG PET/CT can certainly play an impor-ant role in identifying nodal disease in unexpected ocations (upper mediastinum, axilla) and detecting

unsuspected distant metastatic disease. In this setting, PET/CT is advantageous as compared with conventional imaging because of its whole-body coverage and its sensitivity to lesions that might be missed on conventional imaging, such as subtle bone metastases that may not be detectable on a routine chest or abdominal CT scan. Several studies have demonstrated that PET may detect occult distant metastatic disease in as many as 10% of patients with advanced locoregional disease.[11,13,15,17,25] In a prospective study, Chan and colleagues[26] compared the diagnostic value of FDG PET/CT and whole-body MR imaging (WB-MR imaging) for the assessment of distant metas-tases and second primary cancer in 103 patients with untreated oropharyngeal or hypopharyngeal squamous cell carcinoma. On a lesion-based anal-ysis, PET/CT showed higher sensitivity compared with MR imaging (81.0% vs 61.9%, P = .125). On a patient-based analysis, the sensitivity of WB-MR imaging was lower than that of PET/CT (66.7% vs 83.3%, P = .625).

Furthermore, patients with HNSCC have an elevated risk of having a synchronous malignancy, particularly in the upper aerodigestive tract. In a study involving 299 patients with advanced HNSCC, Haerle and colleagues[27] showed a high accuracy of ^{18}F-FDG PET/CT as a screening method for distant metastases in high-risk patients. The sensitivity and specificity of PET/CT in detecting distant metas-tases were 97.8% and 94.8%, respectively. The investigators mentioned that the detected rate of distant metastases either at the time of cancer diag-nosis or during follow-up is considerable and justifies routine screening for distant metastases in patients with advanced HNSCC before extensive curative treatment and during posttreatment follow-up. Also, due to the high accuracy and the one-stage WB assessment, FDG PET/CT is the preferred method for distant metastases screening.

PET/CT is usually recommended when there is concern for distant metastases based on the extent of locoregional disease. If distant metastases are identified, then surgery that would be associated with potential functional loss and morbidity can be avoided. In addition, PET/CT may be used to further evaluate possibly abnormal incidental find-ings from another imaging examination (eg, medi-astinal adenopathy detected on a chest CT scan). A schema for the role of ^{18}F-FDG PET/CT in primary HNC was described by Quon and colleagues[28] (Fig. 2). In their protocol, MR imaging and CT are primary imaging modalities to stage the tumor. PET/CT is only indicated if these methods demon-strate or are suggestive of nodal disease.

A recent multicenter prospective study involving 233 patients supports the implementation of FDG

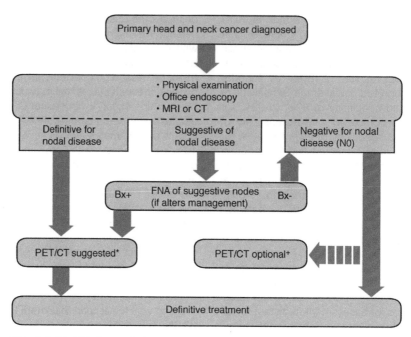

Primary head and neck cancer diagnosed

- Physical examination
- Office endoscopy
- MRI or CT

| Definitive for nodal disease | Suggestive of nodal disease | Negative for nodal disease (N0) |

FNA of suggestive nodes (if alters management)
Bx+   Bx-

PET/CT suggested*   PET/CT optional+

Definitive treatment

*Primarily to detect distant metastatic disease, additional metastatic regional lymph nodes, and synchronous tumors
+Primarily to serve as a baseline prior to therapy

Fig. 2. Algorithm for the initial staging of head and neck squamous cell carcinoma.

PET in the routine imaging work up of HNSCC. The study stated that adding WB-PET-FDG to the pretherapeutic conventional staging of HNSCC improved the TNM classification of the disease and altered the management of 13.7% of their patients (the greater impact was the detection of metastatic or additional disease).[29] Another study involving patients with mucosal HNSCC described that PET/CT had more difficulties in delineating lymph node metastases adjacent to the primary tumor than CT but was superior for the detection of distant and contralateral lymph node metastases. Also, even after a routine clinical staging, PET/CT changed the treatment in approximately 8% of patients.[15] It is important, however, to establish if implementation of PET/CT in the conventional staging will change patient's survival rate.

IDENTIFICATION OF UNKNOWN PRIMARY DISEASE

Approximately 2% to 9% of all HNSCCs present with a metastatic cervical lymph node without clear evidence for a primary tumor site.[30] These patients present both a diagnostic challenge and a treatment dilemma. Treatment consists of radiation therapy directed at the full extent of the pharyngeal mucosa, which may harbor the putative primary site, and is associated with significant

morbidity possibly for little gain. Identification of the primary tumor site is critical because this may identify a site for primary surgical resection or define and limit the extent of radiotherapy.

The initial evaluation for patients with an HNSCC nodal metastasis from an unknown primary should include a thorough physical examination, office endoscopy, and anatomic imaging with MR imaging (or high quality CT) scans. MR imaging and CT scan results may be negative if a primary site is subtle or difficult to separate from adjacent normal structures (like lingual tonsillar tissue), if the primary site is superficial or very small, or if the scan is limited by motion or streak artifact. Multiple studies have assessed the use of PET for detecting an occult primary site, and success rates have generally been at least comparable if not better than anatomic imaging.[31] In a large review of 11 studies by Schoder and Yeung[13] that included more than 300 patients, the sensitivity of PET ranged from 10% to 60%, which was attributed to differences in inclusion criteria and clinical verification. Another meta-analysis concentrated on studies that specifically address the subpopulation of patients that have had an initially negative physical examination and MR imaging. In this group, FDG PET and PET/CT were able to detect the primary tumor in 40 of 150 patients (27%).[32] Rudmik and colleagues[33] did a prospective study comparing CT and/or MR to PET/CT in the etection of the primary site in unknown tumors. They found that CT/MR imaging identified the primary site in 25% of the patients, whereas ET/CT identified the primary site in 55% of the patients. The sensitivity and specificity of PET/CT were 92% and 63%, respectively. The positive redictive value (PPV) and negative predictive alue (NPV) of PET/CT were 79% and 83%, respectively. In a more recent study involving 78 atients with neck lymph node metastases from n unknown primary cancer, a suspicious lesion as found in 59% of the patients. PET/CT diagosed primary cancers in 30 of 78 patients 8.5%); sensitivity, specificity, PPV, and NPV ere 30/30 (100.0%), 32/48 (66.7%), 30/46 5.2%), 32/32 (100.0%), respectively. PET/CT lso detected additional disease in 4 patients: ontralateral nodal disease in 2, mediastinal nodal isease in one, and liver metastases in one.[34]

An indicated protocol is to perform a PET/CT can when physical examination, office endos-opy, and MR imaging are unrevealing.[28] If there s a suspicious focus on metabolic imaging, then ne patient proceeds to panendoscopy, during vhich a frozen section biopsy of the suspicious ite found on PET/CT is done. If the frozen section iopsy result is negative, then further strategic iopsies are obtained from the most common sites or primary tumor. These sites include the base of ongue, the ipsilateral tonsillar fossa, in some ases, the pyriform sinus and the contralateral onsillar fossa, and the nasopharynx. If the PET/ :T does not show any evidence of the primary umor, then patient proceeds to panendoscopy nd subsequent strategic surgical biopsies with ne hope that permanent tissue sections will identify the occult primary tumor. If the primary tumor is discovered, then a PET/CT may be done before treatment to assess for locoregional disease, distant metastases, and a synchronous tumor (**Fig. 3**).

MONITORING TREATMENT RESPONSE AND SURVEILLANCE

Intensity-modulated radiation therapy (IMRT) with concurrent cisplatin chemotherapy is frequently the primary treatment in HNSCC. This nonsurgical treatment may be chosen for either of 2 general reasons. First, an organ-preservation protocol may be chosen in patients with HNSCC in an effort to avoid surgical resection altogether. Second, chemoradiation is often chosen in those clinical scenarios where it has been demonstrated to achieve similar or better locoregional control than protocols that include surgery. In both clinical settings, PET/CT is useful for monitoring treatment response and accurately identifying patients with residual disease for salvage surgery.

Diagnostic uncertainty may result in delayed or unnecessary treatment. Further, the life expectancy and quality of life of these patients may be greatly reduced if not diagnosed properly and in a timely manner. Meanwhile, the assessment of treatment response and surveillance for recurrence in HNSCC may pose a diagnostic challenge. Radiation and surgery can cause significant changes to the normal tissues of the head and neck.[35] Such tissue distortions can obscure persistent or recurrent disease on physical examination, CT and MR imaging until relatively late in the course of disease.[35,36] The conventional structure-based diagnostic tools,

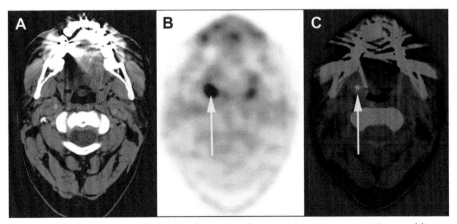

ig. 3. Squamous cell carcinoma neck metastasis from an unknown primary tumor. A 55-year-old man with right eck mass. Fine-needle aspiration showed metastatic poorly differentiated squamous cell carcinoma. (*A*) ontrast-enhanced CT showed only the right neck mass. (*B*) FDG PET and (*C*) fusion PET/CT clearly identifies he primary tumor in the right tonsil (*yellow arrows*), which is confirmed by an endoscopic biopsy and followed y right tonsillectomy.

such as MR imaging and CT, have been proved ineffective in the early detection of residual or recurrent foci for patients with nasopharyngeal cancer.[6,7,37] FDG PET, likewise, suffers from nonspecific increases in tracer uptake in lymphoid tissue, salivary glands, muscles, and soft tissue usually because of posttreatment inflammation.[38] Several studies, however, have shown that PET is more effective than conventional imaging in distinguishing residual and recurrent tumors from posttreatment changes.[39–46]

In a series of 108 patients, Ryan and colleagues[47] found that PET/CT can detect locoregional persistent cancer or recurrent HNSCC with a sensitivity of 82%, specificity of 92%, PPV of 64%, NPV of 97%, and overall accuracy of 90%. Similarly, in a recent report of 39 patients by Porceddu and colleagues,[48] PET had an NPV of 97% when performed at a median of 12 weeks after the completion of therapy. For the detection of distant metastases, PET/CT scans had a sensitivity of 89%, specificity of 97%, PPV of 85%, NPV of 98%, and overall accuracy of 96%.[47] A negative PET/CT scan result is highly reliable for all sites when performed at least 2 to 3 months after therapy (**Fig. 4**).[48] A positive PET/CT scan in the

head and neck region must be correlated wi information from the physical examination ar cross-sectional imaging modalities as nonspeci inflammation may often be FDG avid.

The optimal timing of PET/CT scans relative radiation therapy, once greatly debated, is achievir greater consensus. PET/CT scanning is more acc rate when performed at 2 to 3 months after th completion of radiation therapy than at earlier tim points.[41,48,49] This improvement is attributed subsiding of the nonspecific inflammation ov time. A study demonstrated that PET/CT scans pe formed 3 months after the completion of radiatic therapy had a significantly higher sensitivity ($P<.0$ and NPV ($P<.05$) in the head and neck than scar performed within 1 month.[47] Similarly, PET/CT ha a higher specificity in detecting persistent tum after radiation than contrast CT alone, and the spe ificity for PET/CT was highest when it was performe after 8 weeks of treatment.[47] Other studies hav described similar results with a range of 8 to 1 weeks after the completion of radiotherapy.[41,49,50]

Although it has been proved that PET/CT is a effective tool for HNC follow-up, it is also notoriou for the prohibitive cost. A study assessed cos utility for 3 different strategies in diagnosin

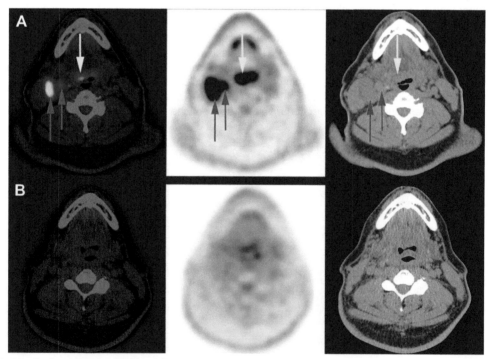

Fig. 4. Monitoring chemoradiation. (*A*) Pre-treatment FDG PET/CT showing an FDG avid primary lesion in th right tongue base where there is soft-tissue fullness (*yellow arrows*) and intensively hypermetabolic right nec mass and jugulodigastric lymph node (*blue arrows*), which were confirmed to be metastatic with biopsy. (*B*) Pos chemoradiation therapy FDG PET/CT demonstrating complete resolution of abnormal activity without evidenc of residual disease in the treated region.

currence for patients with nasopharyngeal ancer after initial chemoradiation: MR imaging-nly, PET-only, and MR imaging followed by PET MR imaging-PET). Under present cost structures f MR imaging and PET, the MR imaging-PET rategy demonstrated to be the most cost effec-ve. They stated that PET-only strategy is still ss cost effective than the MR imaging-PET rategy. However, PET diagnosis is becoming ss costly every year relative to MR imaging, nd PET-only strategy may soon become as cost ffective as MR imaging-PET and may even rpass MR imaging-PET as the most cost-ffective strategy.[45] The investigators also demon-trated that PET diagnosis has higher accuracy 0%) for patients suspected of having residual/ ecurrent HNC from MR imaging results than the ccuracy (70%) for patients without prior MR naging.[45,51]

In the setting of surveillance, numerous studies ave demonstrated that FDG PET/CT has a rela-vely high sensitivity for detecting recurrent isease at the primary site and regional nodal etastases (**Fig. 5**).[52–58] Focusing on those atients who underwent PET or PET/CT at least

12 weeks after all therapy, the reported sensitivity ranges between 93% and 100% for detection of recurrence. Because there may be nonspecific FDG uptake in sites other than malignancy, such as in inflammatory lymph nodes or musculature, the specificity of PET and PET/CT is between 63% and 94%, and additional confirmatory tests should be used when there are abnormal findings.

A protocol for assessing treatment response and surveillance described by Quon and col-leagues[28] suggests that approximately 1 month after the completion of chemotherapy and radia-tion, patients with obvious residual disease or tumor progression are considered for immediate salvage surgery. If there is no clear evidence for residual disease, then the patient is clinically eval-uated 1 month later (2 months after the completion of chemoradiation). Again, if a suspicious site is found on examination, then biopsies are per-formed. Patients who appear to have had a complete therapeutic response undergo MR imaging (or CT if laryngeal cancer). A fine-needle aspiration biopsy is performed if there are suspi-cious areas on cross-sectional imaging. If no evidence of disease is found on physical

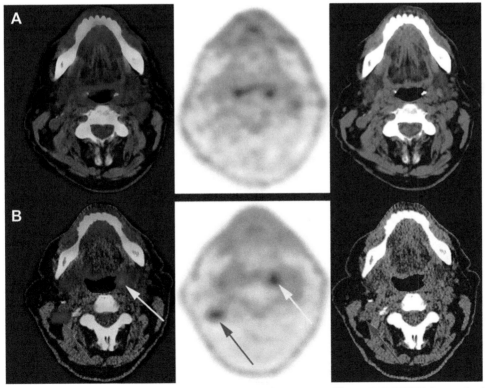

Fig. 5. FDG PET/CT for the detection of recurrence. (*A*) Posttherapy surveillance FDG PET/CT shows physiologic oropharyngeal metabolic activity and mild FDG uptake in subcentimeter, likely reactive, neck lymph nodes without evidence for recurrent disease. (*B*) Interval follow-up FDG PET/CT demonstrates new focal FDG uptake in the left tonsil (*yellow arrows*) and right level II enlarged lymph node (*blue arrows*) concerning for recurrence.

examination, office endoscopy, and MR imaging at 2 months post completion of chemoradiation, then the patient is evaluated by PET/CT beginning at 3 months post completion of chemotherapy. The value of this examination may be increased if a comparison baseline PET scan had been obtained at initial staging. Subsequent surveillance PET/CT scans are scheduled depending either on clinical suspicion or at regular intervals, such as every 6 months for the first 18 months and annually thereafter. In the latter setting, frequent surveillance has a reasonable chance of detecting recurrences and may be of particular value where a potentially curative salvage modality is available (surgery or reirradiation).

RADIOTHERAPY PLANNING

Optimal application of radiotherapy in HNC is challenged by various tumor-related factors: total tumor burden, delineation of the tumor borders, potential damage to healthy tissue surrounding the tumor, and heterogeneously distributed characteristics within the tumor, such as hypoxia and tumor cell proliferation. Advances in radiotherapy such as 3-dimensional conformal radiation, IMRT, image-guided radiotherapy, stereotactic body radiation (SBRT), and proton therapy aim to increase the dose within the tumorous tissue, whereas reduce the dose to the surrounding

healthy tissue. Thus, accurate delineation o tumors and involved lymph nodes has becom very important. Integrated FDG PET/CT imagin provides a bridge between anatomic and func tional imaging that appears ideally suited to radic therapy planning in the era of highly conforma radiotherapy.[59,60] Immobilization devices ar used during the acquisition of the PET/CT sca and improve the registration of PET and CT dat for treatment planning. Several publications repo that target volumes may be modified in as many a 20% of cases when using FDG PET/CT versus C alone (**Fig. 6**). Wang and colleagues[61] stated tha PET/CT was useful for both initial staging an treatment planning in patients with HNC. Patient with a diagnosis of oropharyngeal carcinom may particularly benefit from FDG PET/ CT fusio because it is difficult to identify the oropharyngea tumor by CT scan alone.[61] A more recent study re viewed 96 patients with previously irradiate HNSCC treated with SBRT. PET/CT treatmer planning was used for 45 patients, whereas nor PET-CT planning was used for 51 patients. Cate gories of failure were assigned by comparin recurrences on posttreatment scans to the plar ning target volume from planning scans. PET-C treatment planning was shown to result in lowe rates of failure, particularly near misfailures compared with non-PET-CT planning. The investi gators concluded that PET-CT was advantageou

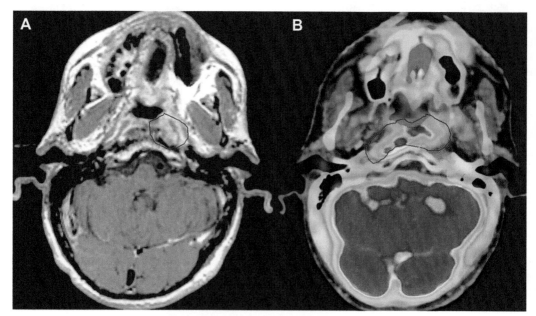

Fig. 6. Using PET/CT to assist in radiation treatment planning. (*A*) MR imaging depicting asymmetric tissue in th left nasopharynx. The radiotherapy contour line is shown encircling this region (*red line*). (*B*) PET/CT showing abnormal metabolic activity crossing midline from the left nasopharynx to the right nasopharynx, suggesting a larger extent of tumor than on MR imaging. The radiotherapy contour is adjusted accordingly (*red line*).

r treatment planning in SBRT for recurrent NSCC, where accurate targeting of smaller mor volumes within previously irradiated tissues critical.[62]

Some investigators have described that PET equently fails to identify hypermetabolism in areas marrow space infiltration and perineural extension at are highly suspicious on MR imaging.[28] Thus, ET/CT primarily is used to include normal-sized, rmal-appearing lymph nodes with increased etabolic activity as part of the high-dose target lume. In addition, PET/CT may be helpful for con- uring primary tumors whose borders are difficult to stinguish by anatomic imaging alone, as is some- nes the case with tongue base tumors. Neverthe- ss, long-term outcome data identifying patterns treatment failure in relationship to PET/CT- gmented target volumes are needed to define standardized approach to using PET/CT in treat- ent planning before PET/CT can be recommended routine practice.

DG PET/MR IMAGING

s mentioned previously, MR imaging and CT rovide accurate anatomic information with high solution. MR imaging provides several advan- ges over CT, such as increased soft tissue ontrast and reduced artifacts close to the skull ase or metallic tooth implants. However, they ave limited sensitivity and specificity, because ey mainly rely on the size criterion. On the other and, FDG PET/CT is sensitive in identifying tumor filtration of the lymph nodes in which neither CT or MR imaging can help distinguish residual or current disease and posttherapeutic changes, ut provides poor anatomic information. Hence,

the possibility of combining different imaging modalities seems promising to minimize the disad- vantages of each method. In general, there are 2 methods available for image fusion: software- based image fusion and hybrid scanners that allow the acquisition of 2 different imaging modalities within a single device and at the same position. These new systems combine the excellent anatomic resolution and high soft-tissue contrast of MR imaging with the high sensitive evaluation of metabolism achieved with PET (**Fig. 7**).[63] A study performed by Lemke and colleagues[64] demon- strated that image fusion is a reliable method to study questionable lesions in liver, pancreas, rectum, neck, and brain tumors. They evaluated 59 MR imaging/PET fusion images and stated that it improves the sensitivity and specificity of the single modality or adds important diagnostic information. A Korean group evaluated CT, MR imaging, ultrasound, FDG PET/CT, and their combined use for the assessment of cervical lymph node metastases in HNSCC. The sensitivity, spec- ificity, and accuracy for MR imaging and PET/CT were 77%, 99.4%, 95.3%, and 81.1%, 98.2%, 95%, respectively. The sensitivity, specificity, and accuracy for combined MR imaging and PET/CT were 85.1%, 99.7%, and 97%. A more recent study evaluated the diagnostic value of fused FDG PET and MR imaging compared with PET/CT, MR imaging, and CT in assessing surrounding tissue invasion of advanced buccal squamous cell carci- noma (BSCC).[65] The sensitivity and specificity of fused PET/MR imaging were the highest among the 4 modalities (90.0%/90.9% for PET/MR imaging, 80.0%/84.1% for PET/CT, 80.0%/79.5% for MR imaging, and 55.0%/81.8% for CT), showing that fused PET/MR imaging is more reliable for

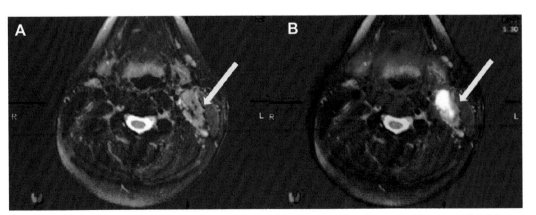

ig. 7. Restaging FDG PET/MR imaging in a patient with widely metastatic salivary gland cancer. (*A*) MR imaging howing a lymph node conglomerate (*yellow arrow*) in the left neck. (*B*) Fusion PET/MR imaging showing hyper- netabolic conglomerate of lymph nodes (*yellow arrow*) in the left neck. (*Courtesy of* Peter F. Faulhaber MD, University Hospitals Case Medical Center.)

focal invasion assessment and tumor size delineation in advanced BSCC compared with PET/CT, MR imaging, and CT.

These publications demonstrated that software fusion of the different imaging modalities performed in separate devices and at different points are feasible. However, authors have described it as time consuming and often limited by different patients positions used for the respective modalities.[66] Many efforts have been made to develop the hybrid PET/MR imaging technology. The major obstacles seem to be the tremendous technical difficulties themselves and the huge cost. Unlike PET/CT systems, new PET/MR imaging designs allow for simultaneous data acquisition. But, the combination of the 2 modalities has a high potential for interference, requiring modification from several sources. Boss and colleagues[63] recently published a pilot study that tested and demonstrated the feasibility of simultaneous PET and MR imaging in the head and upper neck area using a hybrid PET/MR imaging system. They did not observe notable degradation of MR imaging image quality during simultaneous PET data readout. Also, the spatial resolution of the PET component of the PET/MR imaging system was better compared with conventional PET/CT ($\sim$3 mm for PET/MR imaging vs $\sim$5–6 mm for PET/CT), mainly due to the smaller diameter of the PET detector ring and smaller scintillation crystal sizes. They concluded that simultaneous PET/MR imaging of the head and upper neck region is feasible and can be used to obtain complementary information from MR imaging and PET imaging efficiently and with optimal spatial and temporal coregistration. Hybrid PET/MR imaging devices for clinical use have recently been installed and more data are necessary to establish the role of PET/MR imaging in HNC compared with other imaging modalities.

REFERENCES

1. Globocan 2008. International Agency for Research on Cancer; 2008.
2. Siegel R, Naishadham D, Jemal A. Cancer statistics, 2012. CA Cancer J Clin 2012;62(1):10–29.
3. Yeole BB, Sankaranarayanan R, Sunny MS, et al. Survival from head and neck cancer in Mumbai (Bombay), India. Cancer 2000;89(2):437–44.
4. Parkin DM, Bray F, Ferlay J, et al. Global cancer statistics, 2002. CA Cancer J Clin 2005;55(2):74–108.
5. Schwartz D, Ford E, Rajendran J, et al. FDG-PET/CT imaging for preradiotherapy staging of head-and-neck squamous cell carcinoma. Int J Radiat Oncol Biol Phys 2005;61(1):129–36.
6. Chong VF, Fan YF. Detection of recurrent nasopharyngeal carcinoma: MR imaging versus CT. Radiology 1997;202(2):463–70.
7. Olmi P, Fallai C, Colagrande S, et al. Staging and follow-up of nasopharyngeal carcinoma: magnetic resonance imaging versus computerized tomography. Int J Radiat Oncol Biol Phys 1995;32(3):795–800.
8. Sadick M, Schoenberg SO, Hoermann K, et al. Current oncologic concepts and emerging techniques for imaging of head and neck squamous cell cancer. Laryngorhinootologie 2012;91(Suppl 1):S27–47 [in German].
9. Ha PK, Hdeib A, Goldenberg D, et al. The role of positron emission tomography and computed tomography fusion in the management of early-stage and advanced-stage primary head and neck squamous cell carcinoma. Arch Otolaryngol Head Neck Surg 2006;132(1):12–6.
10. Paulus P, Sambon A, Vivegnis D, et al. 18FDG-PET for the assessment of primary head and neck tumors: clinical, computed tomography, and histopathological correlation in 38 patients. Laryngoscope 1998;108(10):1578–83.
11. Goerres GW, Schmid DT, Gratz KW, et al. Impact of whole body positron emission tomography on initial staging and therapy in patients with squamous cell carcinoma of the oral cavity. Oral Oncol 2003;39(6):547–51.
12. Nemzek WR, Hecht S, Gandour-Edwards R, et al. Perineural spread of head and neck tumors: how accurate is MR imaging? AJNR Am J Neuroradiol 1998;19(4):701–6.
13. Schoder H, Yeung HW. Positron emission imaging of head and neck cancer, including thyroid carcinoma. Semin Nucl Med 2004;34(3):180–97.
14. Alberico RA, Husain SH, Sirotkin I. Imaging in head and neck oncology. Surg Oncol Clin N Am 2004;13(1):13–35.
15. Schmid DT, Stoeckli SJ, Bandhauer F, et al. Impact of positron emission tomography on the initial staging and therapy in locoregional advanced squamous cell carcinoma of the head and neck. Laryngoscope 2003;113(5):888–91.
16. Di Martino E, Nowak B, Hassan HA, et al. Diagnosis and staging of head and neck cancer: a comparison of modern imaging modalities (positron emission tomography, computed tomography, color-coded duplex sonography) with panendoscopic and histopathologic findings. Arch Otolaryngol Head Neck Surg 2000;126(12):1457–61.
17. Schwartz DL, Rajendran J, Yueh B, et al. Staging of head and neck squamous cell cancer with extended-field FDG-PET. Arch Otolaryngol Head Neck Surg 2003;129(11):1173–8.
18. Adams S, Baum RP, Stuckensen T, et al. Prospective comparison of 18F-FDG PET with conventional

imaging modalities (CT, MRI, US) in lymph node staging of head and neck cancer. Eur J Nucl Med 1998;25(9):1255–60.

30. Murakami R, Uozumi H, Hirai T, et al. Impact of FDG-PET/CT imaging on nodal staging for head-and-neck squamous cell carcinoma. Int J Radiat Oncol Biol Phys 2007;68(2):377–82.

30. Dammann F, Horger M, Mueller-Berg M, et al. Rational diagnosis of squamous cell carcinoma of the head and neck region: comparative evaluation of CT, MRI, and 18FDG PET. AJR Am J Roentgenol 2005;184(4):1326–31.

31. Hyde NC, Prvulovich E, Newman L, et al. A new approach to pre-treatment assessment of the N0 neck in oral squamous cell carcinoma: the role of sentinel node biopsy and positron emission tomography. Oral Oncol 2003;39(4):350–60.

32. Stoeckli SJ, Steinert H, Pfaltz M, et al. Is there a role for positron emission tomography with 18F-fluorodeoxyglucose in the initial staging of nodal negative oral and oropharyngeal squamous cell carcinoma. Head Neck 2002;24(4):345–9.

33. Schoder H, Carlson DL, Kraus DH, et al. 18F-FDG PET/CT for detecting nodal metastases in patients with oral cancer staged N0 by clinical examination and CT/MRI. J Nucl Med 2006;47(5):755–62.

34. Xu GZ, Guan DJ, He ZY. 18FDG-PET/CT for detecting distant metastases and second primary cancers in patients with head and neck cancer. A meta-analysis. Oral Oncol 2011;47(7):560–5.

35. Teknos TN, Rosenthal EL, Lee D, et al. Positron emission tomography in the evaluation of stage III and IV head and neck cancer. Head Neck 2001; 23(12):1056–60.

36. Chan SC, Wang HM, Yen TC, et al. 18F-FDG PET/CT and 3.0-T whole-body MRI for the detection of distant metastases and second primary tumours in patients with untreated oropharyngeal/hypopharyngeal carcinoma: a comparative study. Eur J Nucl Med Mol Imaging 2011;38(9):1607–19.

37. Haerle S, Schmid DT, Ahmad N, et al. The value of (18) F-FDG PET/CT for the detection of distant metastases in high-risk patients with head and neck squamous cell carcinoma. Oral Oncol 2011;47(7):653–9.

38. Quon A, Fischbein NJ, McDougall IR, et al. Clinical role of 18F-FDG PET/CT in the management of squamous cell carcinoma of the head and neck and thyroid carcinoma. J Nucl Med 2007;48(Suppl 1): 58S–67S.

39. Lonneux M, Hamoir M, Reychler H, et al. Positron emission tomography with [18F]fluorodeoxyglucose improves staging and patient management in patients with head and neck squamous cell carcinoma: a Multicenter Prospective Study. J Clin Oncol 2010;28(7):1190–5.

30. Jereczek-Fossa BA, Jassem J, Orecchia R. Cervical lymph node metastases of squamous cell carcinoma from an unknown primary. Cancer Treat Rev 2004;30(2):153–64.

31. OS AA, Fischbein NJ, Caputo GR, et al. Metastatic head and neck cancer: role and usefulness of FDG PET in locating occult primary tumors. Radiology 1999;210(1):177–81.

32. Menda Y, Graham MM. Update on 18F-fluorodeoxyglucose/positron emission tomography and positron emission tomography/computed tomography imaging of squamous head and neck cancers. Semin Nucl Med 2005;35(4):214–9.

33. Rudmik L, Lau H, Matthews TW, et al. Clinical utility of PET/CT in the evaluation of head and neck squamous cell carcinoma with an unknown primary: a prospective clinical trial. Head Neck 2011;33(7): 935–40.

34. Wong WL, Sonoda LI, Gharpurhy A, et al. 18F-fluorodeoxyglucose positron emission tomography/ computed tomography in the assessment of occult primary head and neck cancers–an audit and review of published studies. Clin Oncol 2012;24(3):190–5.

35. Bronstein AD, Nyberg DA, Schwartz AN, et al. Soft-tissue changes after head and neck radiation: CT findings. AJNR Am J Neuroradiol 1989;10(1):171–5.

36. Laubenbacher C, Saumweber D, Wagner-Manslau C, et al. Comparison of fluorine-18-fluorodeoxyglucose PET, MRI and endoscopy for staging head and neck squamous-cell carcinomas. J Nucl Med 1995; 36(10):1747–57.

37. Ng SH, Chang JT, Ko SF, et al. MRI in recurrent nasopharyngeal carcinoma. Neuroradiology 1999; 41(11):855–62.

38. Goerres GW, Von Schulthess GK, Hany TF. Positron emission tomography and PET CT of the head and neck: FDG uptake in normal anatomy, in benign lesions, and in changes resulting from treatment. AJR Am J Roentgenol 2002;179(5):1337–43.

39. Kitagawa Y, Nishizawa S, Sano K, et al. Prospective comparison of 18F-FDG PET with conventional imaging modalities (MRI, CT, and 67Ga scintigraphy) in assessment of combined intraarterial chemotherapy and radiotherapy for head and neck carcinoma. J Nucl Med 2003;44(2):198–206.

40. Dalsaso TA, Lowe VJ, Dunphy FR, et al. FDG-PET and CT in evaluation of chemotherapy in advanced head and neck cancer. Clin Positron Imaging 2000;3(1):1–5.

41. Andrade RS, Heron DE, Degirmenci B, et al. Post-treatment assessment of response using FDG-PET/ CT for patients treated with definitive radiation therapy for head and neck cancers. Int J Radiat Oncol Biol Phys 2006;65(5):1315–22 [Epub 2006 Jun 5].

42. Klabbers BM, Lammertsma AA, Slotman BJ. The value of positron emission tomography for monitoring response to radiotherapy in head and neck cancer. Mol Imaging Biol 2003;5(4):257–70.

43. Goerres GW, Schmid DT, Bandhauer F, et al. Positron emission tomography in the early follow-up of

advanced head and neck cancer. Arch Otolaryngol Head Neck Surg 2004;130(1):105–9 [discussion: 120–1].

44. Kao CH, ChangLai SP, Chieng PU, et al. Detection of recurrent or persistent nasopharyngeal carcinomas after radiotherapy with 18-fluoro-2-deoxyglucose positron emission tomography and comparison with computed tomography. J Clin Oncol 1998; 16(11):3550–5.

45. Yen RF, Yen MF, Hong RL, et al. The cost-utility analysis of 18-fluoro-2-deoxyglucose positron emission tomography in the diagnosis of recurrent nasopharyngeal carcinoma. Acad Radiol 2009;16(1):54–60.

46. Shu-Hang N, Tung-Chieh JC, Sheng-Chieh C, et al. Clinical usefulness of 18F-FDG PET in nasopharyngeal carcinoma patients with questionable MRI findings for recurrence. J Nucl Med 2004;45(10):1669–76.

47. Ryan WR, Fee WE Jr, Le QT, et al. Positron-emission tomography for surveillance of head and neck cancer. Laryngoscope 2005;115(4):645–50.

48. Porceddu SV, Jarmolowski E, Hicks RJ, et al. Utility of positron emission tomography for the detection of disease in residual neck nodes after (chemo) radiotherapy in head and neck cancer. Head Neck 2005;27(3):175–81.

49. Lonneux M, Lawson G, Ide C, et al. Positron emission tomography with fluorodeoxyglucose for suspected head and neck tumor recurrence in the symptomatic patient. Laryngoscope 2000;110(9): 1493–7.

50. Greven KM, Williams DW 3rd, McGuirt WF Sr, et al. Serial positron emission tomography scans following radiation therapy of patients with head and neck cancer. Head Neck 2001;23(11):942–6.

51. Goerres G, MosnaFirlejczyk K, Steurer J, et al. Assessment of clinical utility of 18F-FDG PET in patients with head and neck cancer: a probability analysis. Eur J Nucl Med Mol Imaging 2003;30(4): 562–71.

52. Fischbein NJ, OS AA, Caputo GR, et al. Clinical utility of positron emission tomography with 18F-fluorodeoxyglucose in detecting residual/recurrent squamous cell carcinoma of the head and neck. AJNR Am J Neuroradiol 1998;19(7):1189–96.

53. Li P, Zhuang H, Mozley PD, et al. Evaluation of recurrent squamous cell carcinoma of the head and neck with FDG positron emission tomography. Clin Nucl Med 2001;26(2):131–5.

54. Lowe VJ, Boyd JH, Dunphy FR, et al. Surveillance for recurrent head and neck cancer using positron emission tomography. J Clin Oncol 2000;18(3):651–8.

55. Hanasono MM, Kunda LD, Segall GM, et al. Uses and limitations of FDG positron emission tomography in patients with head and neck cancer. Laryngoscop 1999;109(6):880–5.

56. Stokkel MP, Terhaard CH, Hordijk GJ, et al. Th detection of local recurrent head and neck canc with fluorine-18 fluorodeoxyglucose dual-head pos tron emission tomography. Eur J Nucl Med 199 26(7):767–73.

57. Terhaard CH, Bongers V, van Rijk PP, et al. F-18-fl oro-deoxy-glucose positron-emission tomograph scanning in detection of local recurrence after radi therapy for laryngeal/ pharyngeal cancer. Hea Neck 2001;23(11):933–41.

58. Wong RJ, Lin DT, Schoder H, et al. Diagnostic an prognostic value of [(18)F]fluorodeoxyglucose pos tron emission tomography for recurrent head an neck squamous cell carcinoma. J Clin Oncol 200; 20(20):4199–208.

59. Ciernik IF, Dizendorf E, Baumert BG, et al. Radiatic treatment planning with an integrated positron emis sion and computer tomography (PET/CT): a feas bility study. Int J Radiat Oncol Biol Phys 200; 57(3):853–63.

60. Heron DE, Andrade RS, Flickinger J, et a Hybrid PET-CT simulation for radiation treatmer planning in head-and-neck cancers: a brief tech nical report. Int J Radiat Oncol Biol Phys 200 60(5):1419–24.

61. Wang D, Schultz C, Jursinic P, et al. Initial exper ence of FDG-PET/CT guided IMRT of head-and neck carcinoma. Int J Radiat Oncol Biol Phy 2006;65(1):143–51.

62. Wang K, Heron D, Flickinger J, et al. A retrospectiv deformable registration analysis of the impact c PET-CT planning on patterns of failure in stereotacti body radiation therapy for recurrent head and nec cancer. Head Neck Oncol 2012;4(1):12.

63. Boss A, Stegger L, Bisdas S, et al. Feasibility c simultaneous PET/MR imaging in the head an upper neck area. Eur Radiol 2011;21(7):1439–46.

64. Lemke AJ, Niehues SM, Amthauer H, et al. Klinische Einsatz der digitalenretrospektivenBildfusion von C MRT, FDG-PET und SPECT - Anwendungsgebiet und Ergebnisse. Rofo 2004;176(12):1811–8 [i German].

65. Huang SH, Chien CY, Lin WC, et al. A comparativ study of fused FDG PET/MRI, PET/CT, MRI, and C imaging for assessing surrounding tissue invasio of advanced buccal squamous cell carcinomɑ Clin Nucl Med 2011;36(7):518–25.

66. Loeffelbein D, Souvatzoglou M, Wankerl V, et al. PET MRI fusion in head-and-neck oncology: curren status and implications for hybrid PET/MRI. J Ora Maxillofac Surg 2012;70(2):473–83.

The Application of FDG-PET as Prognostic Indicators in Head and Neck Squamous Cell Carcinoma

Farzan Siddiqui, MD, PhD[a], Peter F. Faulhaber, MD[b],
Min Yao, MD, PhD[c],*, Quynh-Thu Le, MD[d]

KEYWORDS

• Head and neck cancer • FDG-PET • Prognosis

KEY POINTS

- Fludeoxyglucose F 18 (FDG)-PET can be used to assess the aggressiveness of cancers.
- Its role in serving prognostic information in head and neck squamous cell carcinoma (HNSCC) is being actively investigated.
- Currently no definite standards for its use exist and there is a need to conduct prospective studies to establish such standards.

INTRODUCTION

In the United States, approximately 52,000 new cases of oral cavity, pharyngeal, and laryngeal cancers are diagnosed every year, with approximately 11,000 deaths.[1] Globally, head and neck cancers (HNCs) account for approximately 550,000 new cases each year, with 350,000 cancer deaths, representing 6% of all cancer cases.[2,3] Most HNCs are HNSCCs and often present in locally advanced stages. Treatment approaches include surgery with or without (chemo)radiation or organ and function preserving approach with radiotherapy (RT) or concurrent chemoradiation. Selection of therapy is based on patient and tumor characteristics while trying to achieve a high rate of tumor control balanced with preservation of quality of life of the patient. Prognostic factors can help stratify patients into different risk groups and facilitate selection of treatment approach.

Traditional prognostic factors for HNCs include clinical and pathologic factors, such as tumor stage, presence or absence of lymph node metastases, grade or differentiation, surgical margins, perineural invasion, angiolymphatic invasion, and extracapsular extension of the involved lymph nodes.[4] Some demographic and patient-related factors have also been noted as prognostically significant, such as marital status[5] and baseline quality of life.[6–8] Recently, there has been interest in identifying molecular biomarkers. Human papillomavirus (HPV)–related oropharyngeal cancers have been shown to have a comparatively favorable prognosis.[9,10] Other molecular factors have also been studied; these include p53 mutations,[11,12] vascular endothelial growth factor

Disclosures: The authors declare no conflict of interest with any of the material presented in this article. No equipment, manufacturers, or drugs are discussed.
[a] Department of Radiation Oncology, Henry Ford Hospital, 2799 West Grand Boulevard, Detroit, MI 48202, USA; [b] Division of Nuclear Medicine, Department of Radiology, University Hospitals Case Medical Center, 11100 Euclid Avenue, Cleveland, OH 44106, USA; [c] Department of Radiation Oncology, University Hospitals Case Medical Center, 11100 Euclid Avenue, Cleveland, OH 44106, USA; [d] Department of Radiation Oncology, Stanford University, 875 Blake Wilbur Drive, Stanford, CA 94305, USA
* Corresponding author.
E-mail address: min.yao@unhospitals.org

PET Clin 7 (2012) 381–394
http://dx.doi.org/10.1016/j.cpet.2012.06.003

expression, cyclin D1 amplification, and epidermal growth factor receptor overexpression, all of which have been shown to predict poorer outcomes.[13]

In the past few years there has been an increasing number of studies examining the role of PET and PET/CT scans as prognostic factors for various cancers. In addition to location and size, PET/CT scans provide metabolic and functional information about the tumor. With the widespread availability and use of PET/CT scanners for staging HNSCC, there have been attempts at using PET-derived parameters as quantifiable prognostic factors.

This review addresses the use of FDG-PET–derived parameters as prognostic factors and highlights some of the retrospective and prospective studies conducted in this direction. The challenges faced in incorporating PET-CT parameters for prognostication are discussed and some possible future endeavors to facilitate this type of research suggested.

GLUCOSE METABOLISM AND CANCER

Malignant cells have accelerated metabolism and increased energy production to promote cell survival and fuel cell growth. There is also a need for increased production of precursor molecules that are required for cell division. Therefore, cancer cells have a high rate of aerobic glycolysis with increased activity of enzymes involved in glycolysis. This requires a higher rate of glucose flux into the cells, which is facilitated by glucose transporters (GLUTs).[14–16]

GLUTs are transmembrane proteins that allow the energy-independent transport of glucose across the hydrophobic cell membrane. Thirteen of them have been identified. Of these, GLUT1, GLUT3, and GLUT4 have high affinity for glucose. Glucose transportation across the cell membrane is a rate-limiting step for glucose metabolism. Increased glycolysis in cancer cells is accomplished by increased expression of GLUTs, which results in increased glucose influx. The expression of GLUTs is induced by hypoxia-inducible factor, growth factors, and various oncogenes.[17] Increased expression of GLUT1 has been found in many cancers, including HNC.[17] The level of GLUT expression has also been shown associated with aggressiveness of the cancer. Elevated glycolytic activity and increased expression of GLUT1 are found in more advanced cancer stages and predict significantly poorer treatment outcomes.[18–21]

FDG is transported into the cells through GLUTs with the same mechanism as for glucose and subsequently is phosphorylated by hexokinase.

In contrast to glucose, FDG-6-phosphate cann[ot] be further metabolized and thus accumulates [in] the cells. The amount of FDG accumulated in th[e] cells represents the activity of hexokinase an[d] GLUTs of the cells; thus, FDG-PET can be use[d] as a noninvasive in vivo alternative to estima[te] the activity of glycolysis and GLUTs. Therefor[e,] in addition to detecting and localizing cancer f[or] staging, FDG-PET could be an imaging biomark[er] for assessment of tumor aggressiveness and pre[-] dicting prognosis. FDG uptake in HNSCC ha[s] been shown to significantly correlate with ce[ll] proliferation by flow cytometry.[22,23]

STANDARDIZED UPTAKE VALUE AND OTHE[R] PARAMETERS

To be used as a valid imaging biomarker, accura[te] and reproducible quantification of FDG uptake [is] necessary. The gold standard is measuring th[e] rate of glucose metabolism using a pharmacok[i-] netics model with data obtained from dynam[ic] PET studies. This is not feasible, however, in dai[ly] clinical practice. A simplified measurement usin[g] standardized uptake value (SUV), given by th[e] following formula, is now the most widely use[d] method for the quantification of FDG uptake.

$$SUV = \frac{\text{Tissue activity } (\mu Ci/mL)}{\text{Injected dose } (mCi)/\text{Body weight } (kg)}$$

In this formula, tissue activity is the radioactiv[ity] measured by the PET scanner within a region [of] interest (ROI) or the maximal value; injected dos[e] is the dose of FDG administered, corrected f[or] physical decay. The SUV in this formula represent[s] the activity of FDG within the tumor measured ove[r] a certain interval after FDG injection and norma[l-] ized to the dose of FDG administered and to th[e] body weight.[24]

There are many different factors that can affec[t] FDG uptake and its subsequent quantificatio[n.] The biologic factors include blood glucose leve[l,] interval between injection and PET acquisitio[n,] patient motion and breathing, patient comfor[t,] and inflammatory process near or at the tumo[r.] There are also many technical and physical factor[s] that may affect SUV; these include attenuatio[n] correction, calibration, image reconstructio[n,] data analysis, and so forth, which are beyond th[e] scope of this review and are discussed by othe[r] investigators.[25–28] Despite these factors, it ha[s] been shown that there is a good correlatio[n] between SUV and glucose use rate in variou[s] cancers, including HNSCC.[29]

Various forms of SUV-based parameters ar[e] described in literature. These include

SUVmax—This measures the highest (maximal) SUV in an ROI. It has been the most commonly used parameter in clinical practice because it is believed the most reproducible and independent of how the ROI is defined. It represents, however, only a single point within the tumor/lesion and may not be representative of the entire tumor volume.

SUVmean or SUVaverage—This value may provide a more global picture of the tumor activity because it averages the intensity of uptake in a ROI. It suffers, however, from the subjectivity and variability in ROI definition, which may differ between individuals and institutions.

Metabolic tumor volume (MTV)—This is measured in cubic centimeters and represents the tumor volume with active FDG uptake. There is no standard way for tumor segmentation from PET images (for further discussion, see article 4 on PET in RT treatment planning elsewhere in this issue by Woods and colleagues). Threshold-based method is often used. Some investigators used a threshold of SUV greater than 2.5. Other investigators used 40% or 50% SUVmax as a threshold. The MTV is measured as the tumor volume that has SUV above the selected threshold. The volumes vary significantly, however, depending on the threshold selected (**Fig. 1**).

4. Total lesion glycolysis (TLG)—This is a product of the tumor volume (determined by CT scan or MR imaging) and the SUVmean.

CLINICAL DATA AND REVIEW OF LITERATURE
FDG-PET Obtained Before Treatment

Table 1 summarizes selected studies evaluating the role of pretreatment FDG-PET in predicting treatment outcomes in HNSCC. Most early studies used SUVmax as a parameter because it is simple and easy to obtain. Many studies are single institutional retrospective studies with a heterogeneous population of patients treated with various modalities. Different endpoints were used, including local control, locoregional control, disease-free survival (DFS), or overall survival (OS).

One of the earliest studies, by Minn and colleagues,[30] reviewed 37 patients with HNSCC treated using RT with or without surgery. They found that for patients with SUVmax less than or equal to 9.0, 3-year OS was 73% compared with 22% for those with SUVmax greater than 9.0 ($P = .002$). SUVmax was highly linked, however,

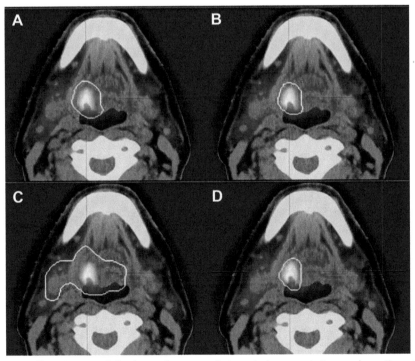

Fig. 1. Squamous cell carcinoma of the base of tongue. Automated segmentation and creation of the primary tumor MTV based on SUV values: (*A*) 40% of max SUV (12.9 mL), (*B*) 50% of max SUV (7.1 mL), (*C*) absolute threshold of SUV 2.5 (77.3 mL), and (*D*) gradient-based algorithm (5.0 mL). Performed on MIM Vista software. (*From* Woods C, Sohn J, Yao M, et al. The application of PET in radiation treatment planning for head and neck cancer. PET Clin 2011;6:149–63; with permission.)

Table 1
Summary of studies on using FDG-PET parameters as a prognostic factor in head and neck cancer

Study/Type	No. of Patients	Sites	Parameters	Treatment	Outcomes (Years)	Conclusions/Significant Findings
Pretreatment						
Schwartz et al,[31] 2004/P	54	Various	SUVmax tumor SUVmax nodal	RT ± CT Sx ± RT		Tumor SUVmax >9.0 → inferior local recurrence-free survival and DFS Nodal SUV → not prognostic
Allal et al,[33] 2004/P	120	Various	SUVmax	RT ± CT Sx ± RT	OS (4)—59% DFS (4)—59% LC (4)—75%	SUVmax >3.5 → poorer LC and DFS
Higgins et al,[36] 2012/R	88	Various HNCs, Opx—66%	SUVmax—primary and nodal SUVmean—primary and nodal TLG	CRT	OS (2)—85% LRC (2)—78% DFS (2)—70%	Increasing primary tumor SUVmean → inferior DFS
Yao et al,[53] 2012/R	284	Various	SUVmax—primary and nodal	CRT Sx → RT	LRC (3)—92.5% Distant metastasis-free survival (3)—84.1%	T-stage and N-stage and SUVnode prognostic for distant metastasis–free survival
Schinagl et al,[41] 2011/P	77	Various	Visual FDG-PET Isocontour SUV 2.5 40% SUVmax 50% SUVmax PET signal-to-background ratio	CRT	LC (2)—84% DFS (2)— 73%	No role for any parameters as prognostic factors
Tang et al,[40] 2012/R	168	Various HNCs, Opx—65%	MTV—primary and nodal	CRT	OS (2)—86% PFS (2)—80%	Total MTV difference between 25th and 75th percentiles increases risk of disease progression and death

Study	Site	No.	PET Parameters	Treatment	Outcome	Findings
Moon et al,[56] 2012/R	Tonsil	69	SUVmax MTV TLG	Sx → RT or RT + CT	90% survival at 28 months	Only TLG predicted for OS
Chu et al,[42] 2012/R	Various	51	MTV velocity based on 2 pretreatment PET scans	CRT—84% RT—6%		1 cm³/wk primary MTV velocity associated with worse outcome
Demirci et al,[57] 2011/R	Various	64	SUVmax	CRT		Nodal SUVmax prognostic for DFS
Querellou et al,[58] 2011/R	Various	89	Tumor SUVmax Tumor/liver SUVmax ratio Tumor/pulmonary artery SUVmax ratio			All 3 parameters prognostic for DFS and OS
Xie et al,[59] 2011/M	Various	1415 in 26 studies	SUVmax			Low pretreatment SUV—better OS, DFS, LC Low post-treatment SUV—better OS, DFS
Murphy et al,[43] 2011/R	Various	47	SUVmax MTV Integrated tumor volume	CRT		Postradiation MTV >18 cm³ prognostic for poorer DFS and OS
Kubicek et al,[54] 2010/R	Various	212	SUVmax	CRT		Primary SUVmax prognostic for OS; nodal SUVmax prognostic for distant recurrence
Liao et al,[60] 2010/R	Oral cavity	347	SUVmax tumor SUVmax nodal Pathologic LNs ±	Sx—45% Sx + RT—27% Sx + CRT—28%		SUVmax tumor—cutoff 8.6 SUVmax nodal—cutoff 5.7 Pathologic LN status— ± Combined scores prognostic for neck control, distant metastasis, disease-specific survival

(continued on next page)

Table 1
(continued)

Study/Type	No. of Patients	Sites	Parameters	Treatment	Outcomes (Years)	Conclusions/ Significant Findings
Inokuchi et al,[52] 2011/R	178	Various	SUVmax tumor SUVmax nodal	CRT	OS (3)—76.5% DFS (3)—58% LC (3)—65%	Nodal SUV ≥6.0→ poorer DFS, nodal progression-free survival, distant metastasis–free survival
Seol et al,[38] 2010/R	59	Various	SUVmax MTV	CRT		MTV >9.3 cm^3→ increased risk of recurrence and death
Machtay et al,[61] 2009/R	60	Various	SUVmax	CRT—62% RT—38%		Pretreatment SUVmax ≥9.0→ poorer DFS and OS
Lee et al,[62] 2008/R	41	Nasopharynx	SUVmax	CRT		SUVmax ≥8→ poorer DFS
Kim et al,[63] 2007/R	52	Oropharynx	SUVmax	Sx→RT CRT		SUVmax ≥6→ poorer LC and DFS
Dobert et al,[64] 2005/R	40	Oral cavity	SUVmax	Chemotherapy→ surgery		Median tumor volume SUVmax = 2.6 in patients with complete response and 5.8 in those with stable disease SUVmax prognostic for chemotherapy response
Halfpenny et al,[65] 2002/P	73	Oral cavity—83% Oropharynx—11% Others—6%	SUVmax	Sx ± RT → 91%		SUVmax >10→ poorer OS

Pretreatment and post-treatment

Study	N	Site	Parameter	Treatment	Outcomes	Results
Moeller et al,[35] 2009/P	98	Oropharynx Larynx	SUVmax tumor SUVmax nodal	CRT	OS (2)—85.7% Disease-specific survival (2)—86.7%	Disease-specific survival correlated with post-treatment primary tumor SUVmax and percent change in primary tumor SUVmax between pretreatment and post-treatment scans Nodal SUVmax → no correlation
Xie et al,[45] 2010/R	62	Nasopharynx	SUVmax tumor SUVmax nodal	CRT	OS (5)—63% DFS (5)—51.6%	Pretreatment SUVmax primary ≥8 prognostic for poor OS and DFS Post-treatment SUVmax tumor with complete metabolic response had better DFS and OS
Inohara et al,[46] 2010/R	31	Hypopharynx	SUVmax	CRT	LC (2)—53% Cause-specific survival (2)—74%	Post treatment SUVmax ≥2.7 → poorer LC and cause-specific survival

During treatment

Study	N	Site	Parameter	Treatment	Outcomes	Results
Hentschel et al,[47] 2011/P	37	Various	SUVmax SUVmean MTV Before RT and 3 times during RT	CRT	OS (2)—51% DFS (2)—44% LRC (2)—55%	Improved OS and DFS for patients with >50% reduction in SUVmax at 10 Gy or 20 Gy

Abbreviations: CRT, radiation therapy + concurrent chemotherapy; CT, chemotherapy; LC, local control; LN, lymph node; LRC, locoregional control; M, meta-analysis; Opx, oropharyngeal cancers; P, prospective; PFS, progression-free survival; R, retrospective; Sx, surgery.

to stage and number of mitoses and thus did not achieve independent prognostic significance on multivariate analysis.

Since this study, several other studies have been published on the role of SUVmax in HNSCC; most used a cutoff point between 5 and 10 (see **Table 1**). Several studies measured SUVmax of the primary tumor (SUV-P) and SUVmax of the lymph node (SUV-LN) separately. Schwartz and colleagues[31] reviewed 54 patients and found SUV-P greater than 9.0 predicted inferior local recurrence-free survival (96% vs 73% for those with SUV <9.0, $P = .02$) and DFS (93% vs 69% for those with SUV <9, $P = .02$). SUV-LN did not show any prognostic significance, however. Yao and colleagues[32] reviewed 177 patients treated with intensity-modulated RT (IMRT). On univariate analysis, SUVmax was not found associated with locoregional control, DFS, disease-specific survival, or OS. On multivariate analysis with SUVmax as a continuous variable, however, SUV-P was significantly associated with disease-specific survival and OS and strongly associated with DFS. SUV-LN was found significantly associated with distant metastasis both on univariate and multivariate analysis.

Although most of the available literature is retrospective in nature, Allal and colleagues[33] conducted a prospective study in 120 patients with HNSCC. Treatment included RT with or without concurrent chemotherapy in 73 patients or surgery with or without adjuvant RT in 47 patients. Pretreatment SUVmax was obtained for all patients and the median SUVmax was 4.76. With a median follow-up of 48 months, 46 patients had recurrent and/or distant metastatic disease. In these patients, the SUVmax was 5.8 versus 3.6 for those patients with disease controlled ($P = .002$). SUVmax remained a significant independent prognostic factor for local control DFS in multivariate analysis.

The SUVmax, however, is significantly dependent on many factors and there are potential limitations for its widespread applicability (discussed previously). This may be a reason that some studies did not show any prognostic significance for SUVmax (see **Table 1**). Vernon and colleagues[34] reviewed 43 patients receiving PET/CT-guided definitive RT and found that neither SUV-P nor SUV-LN was predictive of tumor recurrence. In a prospective study from the MD Anderson Cancer Center, FDG-PET was obtained 4 weeks before chemoradiotherapy and 8 weeks after completion of treatment in 98 patients.[35] SUV-P and nodal SUVmax was calculated for both time points. The only prognostic factor found for disease-specific survival was the post-

treatment tumor SUVmax. Pretreatment SUV- and SUV-LN were not significantly associate with treatment outcomes.

In addition to the limitations of SUVmax (di cussed previously), this parameter represen only a single point within the tumor and may n reflect metabolic activity of the entire tumo Therefore, in recent years, there has been intere in other parameters that may represent a mo global picture of the tumor, such as SUVmea and MTV. The development of sophisticated sof ware for ROI segmentation makes this type analysis feasible and more reproducible.

A recent retrospective study by Higgins ar colleagues[36] evaluated the prognostic signif cance of pretreatment SUVmax, SUVmean, ar TLG in 88 HNSCC patients. The relationship between these parameters for the primary tum and lymph nodes were assessed using a univariat analysis for DFS, locoregional control, and dista metastasis–free survival. The only significar finding was an association between increasin tumor SUVmean and decreased DFS. The 2-yea DFS for those with tumor SUVmean abov the median value was 58% compared with 82% for those with SUVmean below median valu ($P = .03$). A trend ($P = .085$) for poorer locoregion. control with increasing tumor SUVmean was als noted. Neither SUV-P, SUV-LN, nor TLG wa prognostic for any of the clinical endpoints.

Chung and colleagues[37] investigated wheth MTV predicts response to treatment and DFS patients with pharyngeal cancers. MTV was define as the sum of metabolic volumes of the prima tumor and neck nodes, if present. A commercial available SUV-based automated contourin program was used to measure the volume, an a threshold of SUV greater than 2.5 was used define the contouring margins. Using 40 mL a a cutoff, they found MTV predicted treatmer response both in univariate analysis and multiva iate analysis. MTV was also found a significar prognostic factor for DFS both in univariate analysi ($P = .04$) and multivariate analysis ($P = .04$). SUV max of the tumor was determined but not foun associated with either response or DFS. Seol an colleagues[38] likewise used SUV of 2.5 as threshol to obtain MTV and found that MTV was predictive c progression-free survival and OS, but SUVmax wa not associated with either endpoint.

La and colleagues[39] from Stanford Universit also evaluated the prognostic value of MTV in 8 patients. A threshold of 50% maximal intensit was used to define the MTVs. They found tha MTV had a significant relationship with DFS ($P<.001$) and with OS ($P<.001$) on univariate ana ysis. An increase in MTV of 17.4 mL wa gnificantly associated with an increased hazard first event (recurrence or death). SUVmax did ot show a significant relationship with either of ese endpoints, however. A recent report from e same group of investigators validated these ndings in an additional 83 patients.[40] Further- ore, total MTV was also found a significant edictor of locoregional progression ($P = .014$) nd distant metastatic failure ($P = .023$). MTV re- ained a significant predictor in a subset of atients with p16-positive oropharyngeal cancer. hen total MTV was divided into primary MTV nd nodal MTV, only primary MTV predicted rogression-free survival and OS. Nodal MTV pre- cted neither progression-free survival nor OS.

PET-based volumes obtained by different egmentation methods were evaluated by Schinagl nd colleagues.[41] In their study, 77 patients with age II–IV HNSCC treated with (chemo)radiation nderwent pretreatment CT and PET scans. Five ET-based volumes were obtained, including visu- ly delineated PET volume (PET$_{VIS}$) and 4 reshold-based volumes: isocontontour of UV = 2.5 around the tumor (PET$_{2.5}$), volume bove 40% of SUVmax (PET$_{40\%}$), volume above 0% of SUVmax (PET$_{50\%}$), and volume delineated sing an adaptive threshold based on the signal- -background ratio (PET$_{SBR}$). The mean SUV for ach PET-based volume was recorded, which as multiplied by the corresponding volume, re- ulting in integrated SUVs (iSUV$_{VIS}$, iSUV$_{2.5}$, UV$_{40\%}$, iSUV$_{50\%}$, and iSUV$_{SBR}$). They found that hypopharyngeal and laryngeal tumors, none of e parameters was associated with outcomes. In ral cavity and oropharyngeal tumors, PET$_{VIS}$ was ble to predict local control, distant metastasis– ee survival, DFS, and OS, whereas other PET- ased volumes were not. Furthermore, all iSUV ethods were able to predict local control, distant etastasis–free survival, DFS, and OS. It seems e iSUV, a product of volume and SUVmean, is more robust parameter. But SUVmax and SUV- ean had no prognostic value in all subsites for ny endpoint.

From these recent studies, it seems that MTV is better prognostic factor than SUV. This is not urprising because MTV is correlated with the umor volume, which has been shown significantly ssociated with treatment outcomes in HNC. urther studies are needed, however, toward evelopment of better segmentation tools and to etermine which PET-based volume to use. For xample, in approximately half of the patients in e study by Schinagl and colleagues,[41] PET$_{2.5}$ vas not successfully obtained due to significant mount of normal tissue included as judged by isual interpretation. This was not reported in

studies by Chung and colleagues[37] and Seol and colleagues.[38] Also, in the studies by the Stanford group,[39,42,43] MTV was obtained using threshold of 50% of SUVmax. This was not found prog- nostic, however, in the study by Schinagl and colleagues. Instead, they found that MTV obtained by visual delineation was superior. The different segmentation tools they used may be one of the reasons for these discrepancies besides the differ- ences in patient populations. As shown in **Fig. 1**, depending on the threshold selected, the MTV varies significantly, and a consensus is needed for better interinstitutional comparison.

PET Obtained After Treatment

As discussed previously, a prospective study from the MD Anderson Cancer Center[35] showed that the post-treatment SUV-P predicted DFS. The mean SUVmax for those who failed was 7.2 compared with 4.2 for those who did not fail ($P<.01$). Yao and colleagues[44] reported on 188 patients treated with IMRT. The 3-year DFS was 42.5% for those who had a positive post-treatment PET compared with 70.5% for those with a negative PET ($P<.0001$). And the 3-year OS was 57% for those who had a positive post-treatment PET compared with 73.6% for those with a negative PET ($P = .005$). Others have also found post-treatment parameters prognostic.[45,46] The significance of post-treatment PET is discussed elsewhere in article 2 by Mosci and Adams on subsequent therapy evaluation and article 5 on decision making for neck dissection after radiation treatment.

PET Obtained in the Early Phase of Treatment

There are not many studies on the application of PET during treatment, partly because of the cost of repeating PET scans. The clinical implication of obtaining PET scans after starting RT are also not clear as treatments are not interrupted once they start, even though some high-risk patients may be able to be identified. It may be useful, however, in patients receiving induction chemotherapy. But the role of induction chemotherapy in definitive treatment of HNSCC has not yet been defined.

Hentschel and colleagues[47] reported a prospec- tive study evaluated the role of serial PET scans during early phase of RT and the ability of these scans to predict treatment outcomes.[47] In this study, patients were divided into 2 groups and all of them underwent 4 PET scans. In 1 group, PET scans were obtained before treatment, at 10 Gy, 30 Gy, and 50 Gy. In the other group, PET scans were obtained before treatment, at 20 Gy, 40 Gy, and 60 Gy. The investigators found that patients with a rapid early response as determined by greater than or equal to 50% decline in SUVmax at 10 Gy or 20 Gy compared with the pretreatment SUVmax had a significantly higher OS, locoregional control, and DFS at 2 years. The 2-year OS was 88% for those with more than 50% decline in SUVmax compared with 38% for those with less than 50% decline ($P = .02$). The 2-year DFS was 75% and 31% for those with greater than or equal to 50% and less than 50% decline in SUVmax ($P = .1$), respectively. And the 2-year locoregional control rate was 88% versus 40% for those with greater than or equal to 50% decline versus less than 50% decline in SUVmax ($P = .06$). Similar results were obtained when SUVmean was used; more than 40% decline in SUVmean at 10 or 20 Gy compared with pretreatment SUVmax predicted better treatment outcomes.

Kikuchi and colleagues[48] evaluated sequential PET-CT after induction chemotherapy in prediction of pathology response. Sixteen patients underwent PET-CT and MR imaging before and after 1 cycle of chemotherapy, followed by surgical resection. Comparing between pathologic responders and nonresponders, there were significant difference in postchemotherapy SUVmax and percent decrease in SUVmax (both with $P<.001$). A decrease in SUVmax by 55.5% was found the best predictor of pathologic response. None of the MR imaging parameters showed significant difference between the 2 groups. **Fig. 2** illustrates a patient with FDG-PET before and after induction chemotherapy.

Potential Application of Prognostic Indication of PET in the Management of Head and Neck Cancer

Patients with aggressive cancers may need more aggressive treatment. Therefore, identification of prognostic factors may help personalize treatment. For example, HPV-related oropharyngeal cancer has a significantly better treatment outcome. Currently, clinical trails are underway to explore if deintensification in treatment in this patient population is feasible to obtain similar cancer control while reducing treatment toxicities.[49,50] Yet, as shown by Tang and colleagues, even in this patient population, they can be stratified by MTV; those with increased MTV have a significantly poorer outcome. Thus, MTV should be included in stratification in these clinical trials identify those who may have poor treatment outcomes with deintensified treatment.

Roh and colleagues[51] evaluated 79 patients with advanced resectable squamous cell carcinoma the larynx and hypopharynx treated with surgery followed by postoperative chemoradiation therapy (surgery group, n = 40) or chemoradiation with salvage surgery (RT group, n = 39). They reported that patients with pretreatment SUVmax greater than 8.0 had a significantly poorer DFS. When the surgery group was compared with the RT group, the DFS rates were similar in both groups when SUV was less than or equal to 8.0. When SUV was greater than 8.0, however, the surgery group had a better DFS than the RT group although the difference did not reach significant ($P = .085$). The investigators suggested that patients with high FDG uptake may be better treated by surgery and postoperative chemoradiation.

Inokuchi and colleagues[52] reported 178 patients treated with chemoradiation. They found that a high SUV-LN predicted poorer DFS, nodal progression-free survival, and distant metastasis–free survival. They also noted that for patients with SUV-LN greater than or equal to 6.0, those treated with planned neck dissection had better nodal progression-free survival than those without neck dissection. They suggested using pretreatment SUV-LN to select patients for planned neck dissection.

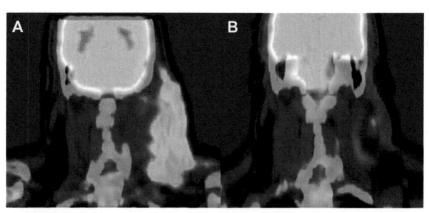

Fig. 2. A patient with advanced squamous cell carcinoma of base of tongue treated with induction chemotherapy. (*A*) FDG-PET obtained before chemotherapy; (*B*) FDG-PET obtained after chemotherapy.

The role of induction chemotherapy in definitive management of locally advanced HNSCC has not yet been defined. As shown by Kikuchi and colleagues,[48] the postchemotherapy SUV and the decrease in SUV after chemotherapy can accurately predict pathologic response to chemotherapy and, therefore, could be used in further clinical trials instead of invasive procedures for assessment of treatment response.

With advanced radiation technique, such as IMRT, concurrent chemotherapy with radiation, and improvement in surgery and flap reconstruction, locoregional control in locally advanced HNSCC has significantly improved in the past decade. Many patients now have distant metastases as their first and only failure. As discussed previously, Yao and colleagues[32] showed that SUV-LN was significant associated with distant metastasis. Recently, the same group updated their experience with 284 patients treated with IMRT and confirmed that patients with distant metastases had a significantly higher median SUV-LN compared with those without distant metastases (11 vs 8.34, $P = .027$).[53] Recent reports by Kubicek and colleagues[54] and Inokuchi and colleagues[52] also showed that SUV-LN was significantly associated with distant metastasis–free survival. Schinagl and colleagues[41] showed that MTV obtained by

visual delineation (PET_{VIS}) and iSUV obtained by various segmentation methods were able to predict distant metastasis–free survival. Patients with high-risk of distant failure benefit from more aggressive systemic treatment either given adjuvantly or neo-adjuvantly. PET-based parameters may help to identify this group of patient in future clinical trials.

SUMMARY AND FUTURE DIRECTIONS

Parameters obtained from FDG-PET can provide prognostic information in HNSCC. Most early studies used SUV-P and nodal SUVmax. The conclusions from these studies were not consistent, however, partly due to the inherent problems in measuring SUV, the heterogeneity of patient and treatment, small patient samples, and the use of different endpoints. In recent years, PET-based tumor volumes (ie, MTV) have been explored and showed more robust than SUV in predicting treatment outcomes. There is need for further development of segmentation tools and for determining which segmentation method can be best applied to the clinical setting.

Furthermore, other prognostic factors should be considered in addition to PET-based parameters. For example, Yao and colleagues[53] showed that N-stage, T-stage, and pretreatment SUV of the lymph node were significantly associated with

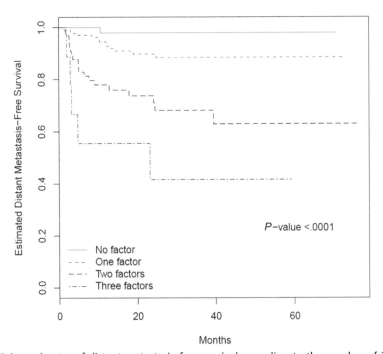

Kaplan–Meier Survival Curve

P-value <.0001

No factor
One factor
Two factors
Three factors

Estimated Distant Metastasis–Free Survival

Months

Fig. 3. Kaplan-Meier estimates of distant metastasis–free survival according to the number of independent risk factors. (*From* Yao M, Lu M, Savvides PS, et al. Distant metastases in head-and-neck squamous cell carcinoma treated with intensity-modulated radiotherapy. Int J Radiat Oncol Biol Phys 2012;83(2):684–9; with permission.)

distant metastasis. The combination of these factors was better than individual factors in predicting distant metastasis–free survival. The 3-year distant metastasis–free survival was 98.1% for no factors, 88.6% for 1 factor, 68.3% for 2 factors, and 41.7% for 3 factors (**Fig. 3**). Moeller and colleagues[35] incorporated HPV status in their mortality risk assessment in addition to post-treatment tumor SUVmax.

The prognostic information from FDG-PET may help in the selection of treatment modality and facilitate personalized treatment. Therefore, PET should be incorporated in clinical trials, especially those conduced by the cooperative oncology groups. The recent completed Radiation Therapy Oncology Group protocol 0522, which compares radiation with cisplatin versus radiation with cisplatin and cetuximab for stage III and IV HNSCC, included pretreatment and post-treatment PET/CT.[55] The results regarding PET are pending analysis. Further collaboration between the Radiation Therapy Oncology Group and the American College of Radiology Imaging Network is important to facilitate prospective incorporation of functional imaging studies in future clinical trials.

REFERENCES

1. Siegel R, Ward E, Brawley O, et al. Cancer statistics, 2011: the impact of eliminating socioeconomic and racial disparities on premature cancer deaths. CA Cancer J Clin 2011;61(4):212–36.

2. Parkin DM, Bray F, Ferlay J, et al. Global cancer statistics, 2002. CA Cancer J Clin 2005;55(2):74–108.

3. Jemal A, Bray F, Center MM, et al. Global cancer statistics. CA Cancer J Clin 2011;61(2):69–90.

4. Bernier J, Cooper JS, Pajak TF, et al. Defining risk levels in locally advanced head and neck cancers: a comparative analysis of concurrent postoperative radiation plus chemotherapy trials of the EORTC (#22931) and RTOG (# 9501). Head Neck 2005;27(10):843–50.

5. Konski AA, Pajak TF, Movsas B, et al. Disadvantage of men living alone participating in Radiation Therapy Oncology Group head and neck trials. J Clin Oncol 2006;24(25):4177–83.

6. Siddiqui F, Pajak TF, Watkins-Bruner D, et al. Pretreatment quality of life predicts for locoregional control in head and neck cancer patients: a radiation therapy oncology group analysis. Int J Radiat Oncol Biol Phys 2008;70(2):353–60.

7. Meyer F, Fortin A, Gelinas M, et al. Health-related quality of life as a survival predictor for patients with localized head and neck cancer treated with radiation therapy. J Clin Oncol 2009;27(18):2970–6.

8. Quinten C, Coens C, Mauer M, et al. Baseline qual of life as a prognostic indicator of survival: a met analysis of individual patient data from EORTC cl ical trials. Lancet Oncol 2009;10(9):865–71.

9. Ang KK, Harris J, Wheeler R, et al. Human papill mavirus and survival of patients with oropharynge cancer. N Engl J Med 2010;363(1):24–35.

10. Gillison M. HPV and its effect on head and ne cancer prognosis. Clin Adv Hematol Oncol 201 8(10):680–2.

11. Koch WM, Patel H, Brennan J, et al. Squamo cell carcinoma of the head and neck in the elde Arch Otolaryngol Head Neck Surg 1995;121(: 262–5.

12. Mineta H, Borg A, Dictor M, et al. p53 mutation, b not p53 overexpression, correlates with survival head and neck squamous cell carcinoma. Br Cancer 1998;78(8):1084–90.

13. Smith BD, Haffty BG. Prognostic factors in patier with head and neck cancer. In: Harrison LB, edit Head and neck cancer: a multidisciplinary a proach. 3rd edition. Lippincott, Williams & Wilkir Philadelphia; 2009. p. 51–75.

14. Vander Heiden MG, Cantley LC, Thompson C Understanding the Warburg effect: the metabol requirements of cell proliferation. Science 200 324(5930):1029–33.

15. Vander Heiden MG, Locasale JW, Swanson K et al. Evidence for an alternative glycolytic pathw in rapidly proliferating cells. Science 201 329(5998):1492–9.

16. Garber K. Energy deregulation: licensing tumors grow. Science 2006;312(5777):1158–9.

17. Macheda ML, Rogers S, Best JD. Molecular ar cellular regulation of glucose transporter (GLU proteins in cancer. J Cell Physiol 2005;202(3):654–6

18. Kunkel M, Reichert TE, Benz P, et al. Overexpressic of Glut-1 and increased glucose metabolism tumors are associated with a poor prognosis patients with oral squamous cell carcinoma. Canc 2003;97(4):1015–24.

19. Zhou S, Wang S, Wu Q, et al. Expression of glucos transporter-1 and -3 in the head and neck carc noma–the correlation of the expression with the bi logical behaviors. ORL J Otorhinolaryngol Rel Spec 2008;70(3):189–94.

20. Roh JL, Cho KJ, Kwon GY, et al. The prognost value of hypoxia markers in T2-staged oral tongu cancer. Oral Oncol 2009;45(1):63–8.

21. De Schutter H, Landuyt W, Verbeken E, et al. Th prognostic value of the hypoxia markers CA IX ar GLUT 1 and the cytokines VEGF and IL 6 in hea and neck squamous cell carcinoma treated b radiotherapy +/- chemotherapy. BMC Canc 2005;5:42.

22. Minn H, Joensuu H, Ahonen A, et al. Fluorodeox glucose imaging: a method to assess th

proliferative activity of human cancer in vivo. Comparison with DNA flow cytometry in head and neck tumors. Cancer 1988;61(9):1776–81.

3. Haberkorn U, Strauss LG, Reisser C, et al. Glucose uptake, perfusion, and cell proliferation in head and neck tumors: relation of positron emission tomography to flow cytometry. J Nucl Med 1991;32(8): 1548–55.

4. Tomasi G, Turkheimer F, Aboagye E. Importance of quantification for the analysis of PET data in oncology: review of current methods and trends for the future. Mol Imaging Biol 2012;14(2):131–46.

5. Boellaard R. Standards for PET image acquisition and quantitative data analysis. J Nucl Med 2009; 50(Suppl 1):11S–20S.

6. Kinahan PE, Fletcher JW. Positron emission tomography-computed tomography standardized uptake values in clinical practice and assessing response to therapy. Semin Ultrasound CT MR 2010;31(6):496–505.

7. Huang SC. Anatomy of SUV. Standardized uptake value. Nucl Med Biol 2000;27(7):643–6.

8. Thie JA. Understanding the standardized uptake value, its methods, and implications for usage. J Nucl Med 2004;45(9):1431–4.

9. Lindholm P, Minn H, Leskinen-Kallio S, et al. Influence of the blood glucose concentration on FDG uptake in cancer—a PET study. J Nucl Med 1993; 34(1):1–6.

10. Minn H, Lapela M, Klemi PJ, et al. Prediction of survival with fluorine-18-fluoro-deoxyglucose and PET in head and neck cancer. J Nucl Med 1997; 38(12):1907–11.

11. Schwartz DL, Rajendran J, Yueh B, et al. FDG-PET prediction of head and neck squamous cell cancer outcomes. Arch Otolaryngol Head Neck Surg 2004;130(12):1361–7.

12. Yao M, Lu M, Savvides P, et al. The prognostic significance of pretreatment SUV in head-and-neck squamous cell carcinoma treated with IMRT. Int J Radiat Oncol Biol Phys 2009;75(2):S17.

13. Allal AS, Slosman DO, Kebdani T, et al. Prediction of outcome in head-and-neck cancer patients using the standardized uptake value of 2-[18F]fluoro-2-deoxy-D-glucose. Int J Radiat Oncol Biol Phys 2004;59(5):1295–300.

14. Vernon MR, Maheshwari M, Schultz CJ, et al. Clinical outcomes of patients receiving integrated PET/CT-guided radiotherapy for head and neck carcinoma. Int J Radiat Oncol Biol Phys 2008; 70(3):678–84.

15. Moeller BJ, Rana V, Cannon BA, et al. Prospective imaging assessment of mortality risk after head-and-neck radiotherapy. Int J Radiat Oncol Biol Phys 2009;78(3):667–74.

16. Higgins KA, Hoang JK, Roach MC, et al. Analysis of pretreatment FDG-PET SUV parameters in head-and-neck cancer: tumor SUVmean has superior prognostic value. Int J Radiat Oncol Biol Phys 2012;82(2):548–53.

37. Chung MK, Jeong HS, Park SG, et al. Metabolic tumor volume of [18F]-fluorodeoxyglucose positron emission tomography/computed tomography predicts short-term outcome to radiotherapy with or without chemotherapy in pharyngeal cancer. Clin Cancer Res 2009;15(18):5861–8.

38. Seol YM, Kwon BR, Song MK, et al. Measurement of tumor volume by PET to evaluate prognosis in patients with head and neck cancer treated by chemo-radiation therapy. Acta Oncol 2010;49(2): 201–8.

39. La TH, Filion EJ, Turnbull BB, et al. Metabolic tumor volume predicts for recurrence and death in head-and-neck cancer. Int J Radiat Oncol Biol Phys 2009;74(5):1335–41.

40. Tang C, Murphy JD, Khong B, et al. Validation that metabolic tumor volume predicts outcome in head-and-neck cancer. Int J Radiat Oncol Biol Phys 2012;83(5):1514–20.

41. Schinagl DA, Span PN, Oyen WJ, et al. Can FDG PET predict radiation treatment outcome in head and neck cancer? Results of a prospective study. Eur J Nucl Med Mol Imaging 2011;38(8):1449–58.

42. Chu KP, Murphy JD, La TH, et al. Prognostic value of metabolic tumor volume and velocity in predicting head-and-neck cancer outcomes. Int J Radiat Oncol Biol Phys 2012;83(5):1521–7.

43. Murphy JD, La TH, Chu K, et al. Postradiation metabolic tumor volume predicts outcome in head-and neck cancer. Int J Radiat Oncol Biol Phys 2011; 80(2):514–21.

44. Yao M, Smith RB, Hoffman HT, et al. Clinical significance of postradiotherapy [18F]-fluorodeoxyglucose positron emission tomography imaging in management of head-and-neck cancer-a long-term outcome report. Int J Radiat Oncol Biol Phys 2009;74(1):9–14.

45. Xie P, Yue JB, Fu Z, et al. Prognostic value of 18F-FDG PET/CT before and after radiotherapy for locally advanced nasopharyngeal carcinoma. Ann Oncol 2010;21(5):1078–82.

46. Inohara H, Enomoto K, Tomiyama Y, et al. Impact of FDG-PET on prediction of clinical outcome after concurrent chemoradiotherapy in hypopharyngeal carcinoma. Mol Imaging Biol 2010;12(1):89–97.

47. Hentschel M, Appold S, Schreiber A, et al. Early FDG PET at 10 or 20 Gy under chemoradiotherapy is prognostic for locoregional control and overall survival in patients with head and neck cancer. Eur J Nucl Med Mol Imaging 2011;38(7):1203–11.

48. Kikuchi M, Shinohara S, Nakamoto Y, et al. Sequential FDG-PET/CT after neoadjuvant chemotherapy is a predictor of histopathologic response in patients with head and neck squamous cell carcinoma. Mol Imaging Biol 2011;13(2):368–77.

49. 1016 R. Available at: http://clinicaltrials.gov/ct2/show/NCT01302834?term=rtog+1016&rank=1. Accessed May 29, 2012.

50. ECOG. Available at: http://clinicaltrials.gov/ct2/show/NCT01084083?term=ecog+1308&rank=1. Accessed May 29, 2012.

51. Roh JL, Pae KH, Choi SH, et al. 2-[18F]-Fluoro-2-deoxy-D-glucose positron emission tomography as guidance for primary treatment in patients with advanced-stage resectable squamous cell carcinoma of the larynx and hypopharynx. Eur J Surg Oncol 2007;33(6):790–5.

52. Inokuchi H, Kodaira T, Tachibana H, et al. Clinical usefulness of [18F] fluoro-2-deoxy-D-glucose uptake in 178 head-and-neck cancer patients with nodal metastasis treated with definitive chemoradiotherapy: consideration of its prognostic value and ability to provide guidance for optimal selection of patients for planned neck dissection. Int J Radiat Oncol Biol Phys 2011;79(3):747–55.

53. Yao M, Lu M, Savvides PS, et al. Distant metastases in head-and-neck squamous cell carcinoma treated with intensity-modulated radiotherapy. Int J Radiat Oncol Biol Phys 2012;83(2):684–9.

54. Kubicek GJ, Champ C, Fogh S, et al. FDG-PET staging and importance of lymph node SUV in head and neck cancer. Head Neck Oncol 2010;2:19.

55. 0522 R. Available at: http://clinicaltrials.gov/ct2/show/NCT00265941?term=rtog+0522&rank=1. Accessed May 29, 2012.

56. Moon SH, Choi JY, Lee HJ, et al. Prognostic value of (18) F-FDG PET/CT in patients with squamous cell carcinoma of the tonsil: comparisons of volume-based metabolic parameters. Head Neck 2012. [Epub ahead of print].

57. Demirci U, Coskun U, Akdemir UO, et al. The nodal standard uptake value (SUV) as a prognostic factor in head and neck squamous cell cancer. Asian Pa J Cancer Prev 2011;12(7):1817–20.

58. Querellou S, Abgral R, Le Roux PY, et al. Prognost value of fluorine-18 fluorodeoxyglucose positro emission tomography imaging in patients wi head and neck squamous cell carcinoma. Hea Neck 2011;34(4):462–8.

59. Xie P, Li M, Zhao H, et al. 18F-FDG PET or PET-CT evaluate prognosis for head and neck cance a meta-analysis. J Cancer Res Clin Oncol 201 137(7):1085–93.

60. Liao CT, Wang HM, Chang JT, et al. Influence pathological nodal status and maximal standardize uptake value of the primary tumor and region lymph nodes on treatment plans in patients wi advanced oral cavity squamous cell carcinoma. I J Radiat Oncol Biol Phys 2010;77(2):421–9.

61. Machtay M, Natwa M, Andrel J, et al. Pretreatme FDG-PET standardized uptake value as a prognost factor for outcome in head and neck cancer. Hea Neck 2009;31(2):195–201.

62. Lee SW, Nam SY, Im KC, et al. Prediction of prog nosis using standardized uptake value of 2-[(18) fluoro-2-deoxy-d-glucose positron emission tomog raphy for nasopharyngeal carcinomas. Radioth Oncol 2008;87(2):211–6.

63. Kim SY, Roh JL, Kim MR, et al. Use of 18F-FDG PE for primary treatment strategy in patients with squa mous cell carcinoma of the oropharynx. J Nucl Me 2007;48(5):752–7.

64. Dobert N, Kovacs AF, Menzel C, et al. The prog nostic value of FDG PET in head and neck cance Correlation with histopathology. Q J Nucl Med M Imaging 2005;49(3):253–7.

65. Halfpenny W, Hain SF, Biassoni L, et al. FDG-PET. possible prognostic factor in head and neck cance Br J Cancer 2002;86(4):512–6.

Radiation Treatment Planning for Head and Neck Cancer with PET

Charles Woods, MD, Jason Sohn, PhD,
Mitchell Machtay, MD, Min Yao, MD, PhD*

KEYWORDS

- PET • Head and neck cancer • Treatment planning

KEY POINTS

- PET is a useful imaging modality in target delineation for radiotherapy treatment planning in head and neck cancer.
- Although there are controversies in some technical aspects, significant advances have been made in image registration and target delineation/segmentation.
- Dose escalation to subvolumes may be possible using PET with FDG and newer tracers that may improve local-regional control.

INTRODUCTION

In 2012, the American Cancer Society estimates that there will be more than 52,000 new cases of head and neck cancers and more than 11,000 deaths caused by head and neck cancer.[1] Most head and neck cancers are squamous cell carcinomas (SCCA), which are the focus of this article. Over the past two decades, landmark studies have led to improved treatments for head and neck cancers and a focus on organ preservation.[2–4] Advances have also been made using chemoradiation postoperatively in locally advanced disease.[5,6] These studies have led to a multidisciplinary approach in the management of head and neck cancers, and radiation treatment plays a central role in the management of head and neck cancer.

Although improvements in survival and locoregional control have been made, the early and late side effects from head and neck radiation treatment continue to be significant. Advances in imaging and computing have allowed radiation oncologists to design more complex radiation treatments. Treatments have moved from 2-dimensional (2-D) plans to 3-dimensional (3-D) conformal planning, and now intensity-modulated radiation therapy (IMRT) is commonly used in the treatment of head and neck malignancies.[7] IMRT, using inverse planning, produces steep dose gradients that allow for highly conformal treatment of tumors while minimizing dose to adjacent normal structures uninvolved by tumor.[8,9] The use of IMRT has led to a reduction in xerostomia and improvements in quality of life following treatment.[10–12] However, highly conformal treatments can lead to disease not being included in the high-dose radiation treatment volume, resulting in locoregional failures. On the other hand, overdrawing the target volumes can result in high-dose radiation being unnecessarily delivered to normal tissues, which may lead to increased toxicities. Therefore, accurate delineation of the tumor volume and regions at risk are critical for achieving the best outcomes.

Advances in computed tomography (CT) and magnetic resonance (MR) imaging have coincided with advances in radiation treatments and are

Department of Radiation Oncology, Seidman Cancer Center, University Hospitals of Cleveland, Case Western Reserve University School of Medicine, 11100 Euclid Avenue, Cleveland, OH 44106, USA
* Corresponding author.
E-mail address: min.yao@uhhospitals.org

PET Clin 7 (2012) 395–410
http://dx.doi.org/10.1016/j.cpet.2012.06.006

commonly used in the design of radiation treatment plans. Although these advances in anatomic imaging have improved our delineation of radiation targets, they give limited information regarding the metabolic activities of tissues and tumor. 18F-fluoro-deoxy-D-glucose (FDG)-PET is being using increasingly in oncologic imaging. Malignant cells have a higher incorporation of the glucose analog, FDG, relative to most nonmalignant cells. Thus, we can exploit this difference to obtain metabolic or biologic information about the tumor and surrounding tissues; however, FDG-PET has limitations. PET has an inherent lower limit of resolution because the positron that is produced during nuclear decay must travel a distance away from the nucleus before it encounters an electron and undergoes annihilation. Also, normal tissues (brain, lymphoid tissue) and physiologic processes (muscle activity, inflammation) can lead to the accumulation of FDG by these cells, making it difficult to differentiate them from malignancy.

Despite these limitations, FDG-PET has proved to be a useful tool in the management of head and neck cancers. Integrated PET/CT scanners are able to provide both functional and anatomic imaging. Initial staging can be accomplished with a single scan that covers most of the body; thus,

simultaneously providing information about the primary tumor, lymph nodes, and potentially metastatic or synchronous disease. PET is now routinely used in the staging of head and neck cancer because of its improved accuracy over CT and MR imaging. Roh and colleagues[13] reported an improved accuracy by PET or PET/CT compared with CT/MR at detecting primary tumors in patients with head and neck cancer (98%–97% versus 86%–88%). Ng and coinvestigators[14] reported improved sensitivity with PET over CT/MR at detecting nodal metastases in 124 patients with oral cavity cancer (74.7% vs 52.6%). Sensitivity was similar between the 2 methods at detecting primary tumor. In a meta analysis by Al-Ibraheem and colleagues,[15] FDG PET or PET/CT was able to detect distant metastases or a second primary in 113 (16%) of 722 patients. Patients can also present with cervical nodal metastases with an unknown primary site of disease. In another meta-analysis of 8 studies, FDG-PET or PET/CT was able to detect the primary site in 51 (28%) of 180 patients with an unknown primary who had a negative initial workup.[15] Accurate staging is the first critical step in treatment decision and treatment planning. **Fig. 1** illustrates a patient with nasopharyngeal

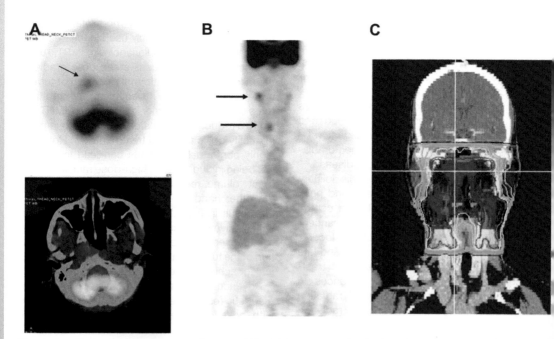

Fig. 1. A patient with nasopharyngeal cancer. (*A*) Initial stage was T1N0 when the patient was referred to our institution after conventional workup. (*B*) FDG-PET revealed hypermetabolic foci in the primary tumor in the nasopharynx and in bilateral level II lymph nodes, which were small and did not meet criteria for lymphadenopathy by CT or MR imaging. Fine-needle biopsies of these lymph nodes were obtained. The right level II node was confirmed to contain metastatic disease, whereas the left level II lymph node was not diagnostic. (*C*) IMRT plan for this patient. The right level II node was treated with a high dose of radiation. The lower neck was treated with an anterior-posterior field.

ncer (NPC) whose level II lymph node was under e size criteria for CT/MRI, but showed FDG otake in the PET scan and was confirmed pathogically. Thus, this lymph node was treated to high dose of radiation.

FDG-PET can also be used to evaluate response treatment. McCollum and colleagues[16] reported n using FDG-PET to assess response to induction nemotherapy (ICT). FDG-PET had a 100% sensirity and 100% negative predictive value (NPV) in etecting residual disease when compared with e gold standard of endoscopic examination and opsy under anesthesia following ICT. Yen and olleagues[17] reported that FDG-PET after ICT can e predictive of outcome in patients with NPC. atients with locally advanced disease were eated with ICT and restaged by PET. Patients no were downstaged by PET were found to ave a significantly improved overall survival ompared with the nonresponder group (33.7 onths vs 44.7 months, $P = .0024$). When assessg tumor response following radiation therapy, Yao nd colleagues[18] reported that FDG-PET had an PV of 98.7% and 99.0% at the primary tumor te and cervical nodal sites respectively. Gupta nd coinvestigators[19] performed a meta-analysis f 51 studies involving 2335 patients to evaluate ET performance for posttreatment response. The ooled PPV and NPV were 52.1% and 94.5% espectively. PET demonstrates a high NPV and negative posttreatment PET is highly suggestive f the absence of viable disease and can be helpful posttreatment patient management decisions.

PET imaging can also be a powerful tool for rget delineation of tumors in treatment planning nd has been increasingly incorporated into daily ractice by radiation oncologists. In a random urvey of radiation oncologists conducted by impson and colleagues,[20] 95% of respondents eported using advanced imaging for target delination with FDG-PET being the most commonly sed (76%). The goal of this article was to explore ow PET is currently being used in radiation treatnent planning and to highlight areas that may enefit from further study.

IMAGE REGISTRATION

efore determining target volumes for IMRT planing, treatment planning CT and PET data must be oregistered accurately. Ideally, a dedicated PET/ reatment planning CT would be obtained at the ame time, in the treatment position with the atient immobilized with a thermoplastic mask so s to minimize patient movement. However, nost radiation oncology facilities do not have dedicated PET/CT scanner and patients often

have PET or PET/CT scans as part of their diagnostic and staging workup before meeting with the radiation oncologist. Patients are often unable to have a second PET scan for treatment planning because of insurance restrictions. PET data, therefore, is most frequently obtained with the patient in a different head/neck position, without an immobilization mask, and lying on a curved table. Therefore, we need accurate methods for aligning the PET with the treatment planning CT scan. Most commercial treatment planning systems offer rigid registration, which can be performed manually or with the aid of an automated algorithm. More recently, algorithms have been developed that perform nonrigid registration and deform one set of images to align with the other. Theoretically, this can lead to better registration of tumor and normal tissue volumes between the PET and CT data.

Schwartz and colleagues[21] at the University of Washington used a nonrigid algorithm developed by Mattes and colleagues[22] for use in an institutional protocol examining the use of a pre–radiation therapy PET and planning CT for head and neck radiation. Images for both PET and CT were acquired with the patient in a thermoplastic immobilization mask. They reported that validation studies of this nonrigid algorithm showed a mean registration error in the range of 0.0 to 2.8 mm (SD 2.8–5.6 mm).

Vogel and colleagues[23] studied various methods of coregistration, including automated algorithm-based methods and manual methods. They reported that the most accurate method was a landmark-based system in which 4 multimodality fiducials detectable by the PET and CT scanners are placed on the treatment planning mask and manually aligned, followed by an automated algorithm that seeks to minimize the registration error. The disadvantages of such a method include the need for multiple fiducials and the relatively longer length of time that is required to produce the coregistration.

Two groups have reported comparison studies of rigid and nonrigid registration for head and neck cancers. Ireland and colleagues[24] studied 5 patients who underwent a treatment planning CT scan and also 2 PET/CT scans: one with a thermoplastic immobilization mask on a flat table (treatment position) and another without a mask and on a curved table (diagnostic position, what one would most commonly encounter in practice). Each PET/CT was registered with the treatment planning CT using either an automated rigid or nonrigid algorithm. The accuracy of each registration method was determined by 4 independent observers who chose 5 landmarks on both planning CT and registered CT. The distance between these 2 points was calculated and reported as a root mean square (RMS) value. They observed that for patients who had a PET/CT obtained in the treatment position, the RMS error for nonrigid registration was significantly less than for patients that underwent rigid registration (2.77 mm vs 4.96 mm, $P = .001$). The improvement with nonrigid registration was even evident with patients who had a PET/CT in a diagnostic position (3.20 mm vs 5.96 mm, $P<.001$). Moreover, nonrigid registration with diagnostic position images were more accurate than rigid registration with treatment position images (3.20 mm vs 4.96 mm, $P = .012$).

Hwang and colleagues[25] reported on 12 patients and compared various methods of rigid registration with nonrigid registration. In this comparison, patients had PET/CT and a treatment planning CT performed. Three of the patients had their PET/CT scan in the treatment position on a flat table in an immobilization mask. PET data were also separated from the PET/CT data for an analysis of PET:-treatment planning CT registration and PET/CT:treatment planning CT registration. PET/CT data were registered to the planning CT using 1 of 3 methods: manual rigid, automated rigid algorithm, and a commercially available (MIM Vista, Cleveland, Ohio) nonrigid algorithm. The standalone PET data were registered to the planning CT using an automated rigid algorithm. Tumor and normal structure contours were then delineated on the PET or PET/CT and then transferred to the planning CT. An analysis was performed by assessing the overlap of normal structures and was reported as a Dice similarity coefficient (DSC). An analysis of the distance between the centers of mass (COM) of the volumes was also reported. Hwang and coinvestigators[25] reported that nonrigid registration resulted in the best registration for brain, spinal cord, and mandible compared with all of the rigid registration methods as assessed by DSC. When assessed by distance from COM, the nonrigid registration was superior to automated rigid registration (1.1 mm vs 4.5 mm for the brain, $P<.001$ and 5.3 mm vs 10.6 mm for the spinal cord, $P<.001$). The investigators noted that nonrigid registration was less accurate in correctly defining the brainstem likely because of its lack of high contrast borders and the chosen algorithm. Three patients had a PET/CT performed in the treatment position and the accuracy of registration was improved, as expected. Together, these 2 studies demonstrate that nonrigid algorithms result in a more accurate image registration and that PET/CT obtained in the treatment position is superior to PET/CT obtained in a diagnostic manner.

At our institution, patients undergo a treatment planning CT while immobilized in a thermoplastic head/shoulder mask on an IMRT board. Patients then undergo a PET/CT scan in nuclear medicine in the same mask in the treatment position on the IMRT board under the supervision of a radiation therapist. We then use our in-house software developed for rigid and deformable image registration to perform registration of the PET/CT and treatment planning CT data. Because the human body is not a rigid object, perfect matching of the 2 image sets is not possible. Therefore, we should compromise the accurate matching over the entire image set or selected area. For the rigid registration, we formulate Spatially Weighted Mutual Information (SWMI) image registration with Structure-of-Interest (SOI)-based weight function (SWMI-SOI) because assigning various importance weight values to geometric location is not possible with mutual information image registration.[26] The SWMI method allows the user to assign the importance weights through the geometric space. The user can choose how much importance weight will be assigned to each SOI as illustrated in **Fig. 2**. We assign the higher importance value to clinical target volume and the organ-at-risk volumes. The highest importance value is often assigned to the volumes that are delineated using PET segmentation tools. Lower-weight values are assigned to other structures so that they will not dominate the registration. This ensures PET-defined volumes will get a full treatment dose in every fraction. Our in-house system also allows the user to assign rigid or deformable (2-D and 3-D affine, or b-spline) image registration to each SOI.

TARGET VOLUMES

Several groups have investigated changes in target volumes with the use of FDG-PET data. Ciernik and colleagues[27] reported on target volume changes when volumes were delineated based on PET/CT versus CT alone. Thirty-nine patients were included in the study with 12 having head and neck cancer. Patients were immobilized and imaged in an integrated PET/CT scanner. PET and CT data were coregistered in the treatment planning system. A radiation oncologist first contoured the gross tumor volume (GTV) using the CT data with the aid of any MR imaging data that were available, and then delineated the areas of suspected tumor involvement with the CT overlayed with PET using a visual method. In the group with head and neck cancer, they noted that the use of PET/CT data for target delineation changed the volume by 25% or more for half of the patients

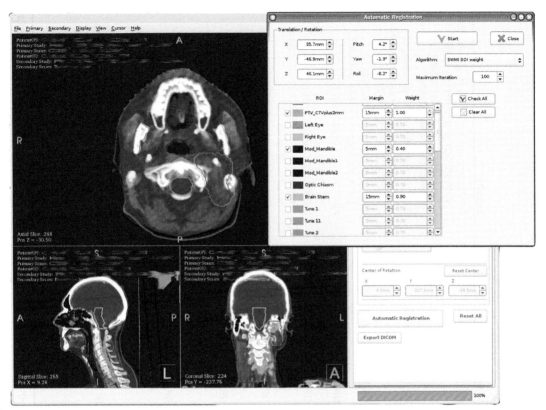

Fig. 2. Two CT images are fused by using our SWMI-SOI automatic registration algorithm. Importance weight can be assigned to each structure-of-interest by a user. (*From* Woods C, Sohn J, Yao M. The Application of PET in Radiation Treatment Planning for Head and Neck Cancer. PET Clinics 2011;6:152; with permission.)

studied. Using PET data resulted in a decrease in the target volume in one-third of patients. The mean GTV change was 32%, which resulted in a planning target volume (PTV) change of 20%. For all cancer sites, they also reported a decrease in interobserver variability. The mean volume difference between the 2 delineation methods was 26.6 mL with CT planning and 9.1 mL with PET/CT planning ($P = .02$).

Paulino and colleagues[28] also examined how target volumes change with the addition of PET data. Forty patients with head and neck cancer underwent IMRT planning. Patients underwent a contrasted treatment planning CT and PET/CT scans in the treatment position. The treatment planning CT was coregistered with the CT data from the PET/CT. GTVs using PET were delineated using a 50% standardized uptake value (SUV) intensity level relative to tumor maximum. They found that the median CT-based GTV was 37.2 mL compared with 20.3 mL with the PET-based GTV. The PET-GTV was smaller in 75% of the cases, with the largest difference being a CT-GTV-to-PET-GTV ratio greater than 5.0 in 7 patients. The PET-GTV was larger than CT-GTV

in 7 patients. Furthermore, in some patients, the PET-GTV was not completely within the CT-GTV even though the PET-GTV was smaller than or the same size as CT-GTV. When 7-field IMRT plans were designed based on the CT-GTVs, the volume of the PET-GTV receiving at least 95% of the prescribed dose was less than 95% in a quarter of the cases. The investigators suggested using the combined CT-GTV and PET-GTV for dose prescription.

Deantonio and coinvestigators[29] studied 22 patients and compared GTVs derived from CT alone, PET, and PET/CT. The investigators used a threshold of 40% of the tumor maximum SUV to delineate PET-GTVs. They found no significant difference in volumes obtained from PET or CT alone; however, volumes contoured from PET/CT data were significantly larger when compared with CT alone (26 mL vs 20 mL, $P<.001$). They also reported that the use of PET resulted in a TMN stage change in 22% of patients.

Several authors[27–35] have investigated changes in GTV when PET data are incorporated into defining target volumes. The results of these studies are summarized in **Table 1**. There is a trend

Table 1
Summary of studies reporting changes in the GTV with the addition of PET data

Author Year	No. Patients	Segmentation Method	Contrasted CT	Comparison	Sites Studied	Stage	Results
Ciernik et al,[27] 2003	12 H&N/39	Visual	No	CT vs PET/CT	NR	IIB-IVA	GTV increased by ≥25% in 2 patients with PET/CT Decreased by ≥25% in 4 patients. PET/CT decreased interobserver variability
Guido et al,[30] 2009	38	50% of max SUV	Yes	CT vs PET/CT	OP NP L HPPNS SG	I-IVB	GTV decreased in 92% of cases; increased in 8% of cases; resulted in stage change in 6/38 cases
Paulino et al,[28] 2005	40	50% of max SUV	Yes	CT vs PET	OP NP PNS L HP OC SG	95% III-IV	PET-GTV was smaller in 75% of patients, larger in 18% patients
Scarfone et al,[31] 2004	6	50% of max SUV	No	CT vs PET/CT	NR	NR	PET/CT-GTV larger than GTV-CT in all cases
Deantonio et al,[29] 2008	22	40% max SUV	No	CT vs PET/CT	OP OC HP L NP PNS	I-IVB	PET/CT-GTV larger in 86% of cases, same size in 14%; stage changed in 22% of cases
El-Bassiouni et al,[32] 2007	25	Visual	No	CT vs PET/CT	OP NP PNS HP L OC	I-IV	Mean CT-GTV significantly larger than PET-GTV. Larger in 72% of cases, smaller in 28% of cases
Henriques de Figueiredo et al,[33] 2009	9	Automated, source-to-background method	Yes	CT vs PET	NR	NR	Mean PET-GTV significant smaller than GTV-CT. Mean difference 40 mL
Wang et al,[34] 2006	28 16 (GTV comparison)	SUV >2.5	Yes	CT vs PET/CT	NP OP HP OC L	II-IVb	CT-GTV larger in 9/27 patients; smaller in 5/28 patients; mean percent change in volume 9.24% (CT larger); changed staging in 57% of cases
Heron et al,[35] 2004	19 H&N/21	Visual	Yes	CT vs PET	NP OP OC L HP PNS	II-IV	PET-GTV mean 42.7 vs CT-GTV 65 mL, $P = .002$; average ratio 3.1; Detected unknown primary in 3 cases and metastatic disease in 3 cases

Abbreviations: CT, computed tomography; GTV, gross tumor volume; H&N, head and neck; HP, hypopharynx; L, larynx; NP, nasopharynx; NR, not reported; OC, oral cavity; OP, oropharynx; PNS, paranasal sinus; SG, salivary gland; SUV, standardized uptake value.

r decreasing GTVs when PET data alone are sed for contouring. If the PET and CT data are sed in conjunction, the GTV is usually larger an with CT alone. Furthermore, the changes in TV vary widely and likely reflect the different xperiences of the investigators as well as whether not contrast was used in the CT scan and the arious methods of segmentation to delineate e edge of the tumor.

EGMENTATION

wing to the inherent spatial resolution limits of ET technology, tumor borders on a PET image ppear blurred. As discussed previously, several vestigators have compared GTVs obtained with e aid of PET with those with CT alone. There is ide variability in GTV volumes between these tudies that, in part, stem from the segmentation ethod used in interpreting the PET data. In other ords, variability may result from how the investi-ators define the edge of the PET tumor volume. A sual method in which a radiation oncologist or uclear medicine physician manually adjusts the indow level is often used by clinicians; however, is method is highly subjective. At what SUV level o we call something disease versus uninvolved ssue? Several investigators have compared ifferent segmentation methods in an attempt to nswer this question.

Schinagl and colleagues[36] compared GTVs from DG-PET using 5 different segmentation methods ith GTV delineated from contrasted CT with the id of other available imaging, such as MR imaging nd physical examination. The 5 methods explored ere the following: a visual method, SUV 2.5 iso-ontour, 40% and 50% threshold of maximum umor SUV (SUVmax), and an adaptive threshold ased on the signal-to-background ratio that was pecific for each case. Seventy-eight patients ere included in the study. In 1 patient, the tumor as not visualized on PET. Schinagl and col-eagues[36] reported that using a SUV 2.5 isocontour esulted in tumor volumes that were overly large, which resulted in unsatisfactory volumes in 35 atients. The GTV obtained from the visual method as similar in size to the GTV obtained by CT alone. Mean volumes were 21.5 and 22.7 mL respectively. he 3 threshold-based segmentation methods all roduced significantly smaller volumes than those erived from CT alone. The mean volumes for the 0% SUVmax, 50% SUVmax, and adaptive hresholds were 16.4, 10.5, and 11.2 mL respec-vely. They also examined the amount of overlap etween GTVs from CT and those from FDG-PET nethods. All methods resulted in significant mounts of PET-GTV volume outside of the CT-

GTV. The 50% of maximum SUV threshold and the adaptive threshold based on signal-to-background ratio resulted in the lowest volume of PET-GTV outside of the CT-GTV.

Greco and colleagues[37] also compared different segmentation methods. For 12 patients with locally advanced head and neck cancer, a reference GTV was defined on a noncontrasted CT scan with the aid of MR imaging data. Patients also underwent a PET/CT scan and the PET data were registered with the treatment CT scan. PET-GTVs were then defined using the following methods: visual inspection, an absolute SUV threshold of 2.5, 50% of maximum SUV, and an iterative segmentation algorithm. Mean tumor volumes obtained from each method were 75.5, 57.6, 60.0, 16.8, and 26.1 mL for CT, visual inspection, absolute SUV 2.5, 50% of maximum threshold, and iterative algo-rithm, respectively. The visual and absolute threshold SUV 2.5 did not result in statistically significant different volumes when compared with the GTV defined by CT. The volumes derived from 50% of maximal SUV threshold or the iterative algorithm resulted in smaller volumes when compared with CT-GTV in all cases.

At our institution, our in-house software uses an adaptive threshold based on the signal-to-background (S/B) ratio. Daisne and colleagues[38] considered the relationship between S/B ratio and iso-activity level for volume segmentation. Their method provides the better accuracy for small and/or poorly contrasted lesions. Our soft-ware calculates the S/B ratio and allows the user to define interactively using a mouse by drawing a line from the highest density to the lowest signal area, as shown in **Fig. 3**. Initially, our software automatically decides the threshold by consid-ering S/B ratio estimation. Then, contours for the tumor volumes are generated by region growing algorithm.[39] The software has an option for the user to change the threshold.

PATHOLOGY CORRELATION

To better understand the optimal SUV values for GTV delineation using PET data, some investigators have correlated GTVs with pathologic specimens. Comparison of PET-GTVs with CT-GTVs has limited value unless it is in the context of pathology and true disease. When interpreting these reports, it is important to note how the tissue was processed for pathology. Fixation with formalin-based methods can lead to significant tissue shrinkage, which has been shown to cause stage migration in patients with non–small cell lung cancer.[40]

Burri and coinvestigators[41] correlated GTVs derived from different segmentation methods

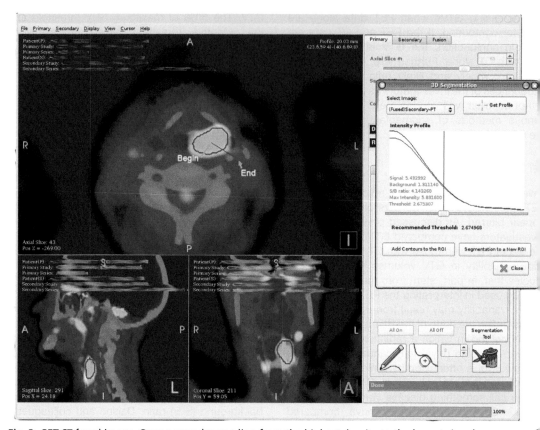

Fig. 3. PET:CT fused image. Once a user draws a line from the highest density to the lowest signal area, our sof ware calculates the S/B ratio and determines the appropriate threshold. The user can interactively modify th parameters in the 3-D segmentation pop-up window if necessary. (*From* Woods C, Sohn J, Yao M. The Applicatio of PET in Radiation Treatment Planning for Head and Neck Cancer. PET Clinics 2011;6:157; with permission.)

using SUV from PET scans with pathologic speci-mens. They studied 28 tumors in 18 patients with head and neck cancers. Surgical specimens were processed in a formalin-based manner. A nuclear medicine physician defined a GTV based on CT and PET using predefined SUV cutoff models: default software window (SUVdef), source-to-background method in which the limits of the window were decreased by 1 SD (SUV-1SD), a threshold of SUV greater than or equal to 2.5 (SUV2.5), or a threshold of 40% (SUV40) of maximum SUV. They reported that PET was supe-rior to CT for detecting primary tumors with a sensi-tivity of 94% and 82%, respectively, and superior for staging of the neck with a sensitivity of 90% and 67%, respectively. Specificity for staging of the neck was 78% for both PET and CT. Pathology data were available for 12 tumors. The SUV2.5 and SUV40 methods of defining GTV were the most likely to overestimate tumor volume, but, impor-tantly, were also the least likely to underestimate tumor volume. SUVdef and SUV-1SD methods tended to overestimate less but also led to

a greater underestimation of tumor volumes tha clinically could lead to treatment failure. The inves tigators concluded that the threshold cutoff c 40% of maximum SUV was the best delineatio method. This study showed excellent sensitivit of PET/CT in the ability to detect tumor an suggests that using an SUV threshold of 40% c maximal SUV may be ideal for creating GTV However, tumor volumes may have been signif cantly smaller owing to formalin processing, whic introduces error to the correlation.

Daisne and colleagues[42] reported on th pathology correlation of CT, PET, and MR imagin in patients with SCCA of the oropharynx, hypc pharyx, or larynx. Surgical specimens were prc cessed in a gelatin solution to minimize tissu shrinkage. Patients underwent CT, MR imagin and PET scans and 1 investigator delineate GTVs based on MR and CT. PET-GTV was autc matically delineated using an S/B ratio algorithm Of the 29 patients included in the study, 9 patient had a surgical specimen for comparison. Fc oropharyngeal tumors, the GTVs contoured usin

T or MR imaging were significantly larger (73% nd 64% respectively) than GTVs contoured on ET. No significant differences were noted etween MR and CT contours. No contours were oted to have total overlap. Similar results were oted for hypopharyngeal and laryngeal tumors. When GTVs were compared with surgical specimens from laryngectomies of 9 patients, the mean GTVs from CT (20.8 mL), PET (16.3 mL), and MRI (23.8 mL) were significantly larger than the surgical specimen (12.6 mL). All modalities resulted in overestimation of tumor volume; PET resulted in the lowest, with 46% overestimation. It was noted that all modalities underestimated superficial tumors.

Seitz and colleagues[43] used pathology correlation to compare GTVs delineated from PET/CT and MR imaging. They studied 66 patients with oral or oropharyngeal cancer, 25 of them with recurrent disease. Pathology specimens were prepared in a gelatin solution to minimize shrinkage. For PET, GTVs of the primary tumor were delineated automatically using an SUV threshold of 3.5. MR imaging GTVs were delineated by 2 senior radiologists using a set of predetermined criteria. There were no statistically significant differences between the 2 modalities at detecting disease. The specificity of correctly detecting the primary disease with MR imaging and PET/CT was 100% and 96.7% respectively. Both modalities detected all primary tumors in patients with recurrent disease. For detecting nodal disease, MR imaging and PET/CT had a sensitivity/specificity of 88.3%/84.0% and 83.8%/74.0% respectively. The mean GTVs from pathology, MR imaging, and PET/CT were 16.6, 17.6, and 18.8 mL, respectively. These differences among the 3 methods were statistically significant. MR imaging and PET/CT overestimated the T stage in 18% and 22% of cases, respectively. More clinically relevant to tumor control, both modalities underestimated T stage, in 8% and 12% of cases, respectively. They found no difference in the detection of the primary tumor by MR or PET/CT, and overestimation and underestimation of T stage were similar between the 2 modalities. This study differs from the results of Daisne and coinvestigators,[42] who showed that PET resulted in a smaller GTV than MRI. However, the investigators studied different disease sites and used different segmentation methods to delineate PET volumes.

Absolute threshold and percentages of maximum SUV are more straightforward to apply to treatment planning, but new algorithms taking into account S/B ratio and how rapidly the signal falls off are being developed to delineate the edge of the tumor volume. Geets and colleagues[44]

reported on a gradient-based method for image segmentation. They analyzed this method in 7 patients with T3 or T4 laryngeal cancer who underwent layngectomy and compared the results with those obtained by an adaptive threshold–based method described by Daisne and colleagues[38] in which an appropriate threshold is chosen based on the S/B ratio of a particular case.[44] GTVs obtained by both PET segmentation methods were compared with surgical specimens that were frozen and sectioned for analysis (nonformalin-based method). The investigators found that the gradient-based method dramatically reduced the overestimation of the macroscopic tumor volume compared with the adaptive threshold method but led to a larger average false-negative volume. The correlation between the gradient-based method and the pathology specimens were better when compared with the adaptive threshold–based method.

Murphy and coinvestigators[45] studied the tumors of 23 patients with SCCA of the oral cavity and explored a variety of segmentation techniques, including absolute threshold, relative threshold, and gradient algorithms. A formalin-based method was used with the average decrease in tumor length from fixation being 14%. The investigators demonstrated relatively poor correlations (R^2 range 0.29–0.58) with the different segmentation techniques; however, this correlation improved with the addition of tumor grade and maximum SUV data. The investigators hypothesized that the underlying tumor biology (eg, grade) influences FDG uptake and may be key in determining the optimal SUV threshold for accurate segmentation.

Zaidi and colleagues[46] analyzed 9 different PET segmentation techniques[47] in 7 patients who underwent total laryngectomy. Laryngectomy specimens were resected "en bloc" and fixed in a gelatin solution, cut, and digitized for 3-D reconstruction. Five threshold techniques, a level set technique, stochastic expectation maximization approach, fuzzy clustering-based segmentation (FCM), and spatial wavelet–based FCM were tested for correlation with the 3-D digitized tissue specimen. The most accurate segmentation technique was the spatial wavelet-based FCM, which underestimated the tumor volume by 6% on average.

Fig. 4 demonstrates how GTV volumes can differ in a patient with SCCA of the base of the tongue, according to which segmentation method is used to define the edge of the primary tumor. GTVs varied from 20 mL to 40 mL depending on the method used. An absolute threshold of 2.5 resulted in a volume that included uninvolved tissue in the soft palate, which would not be appropriate for radiation treatment planning.

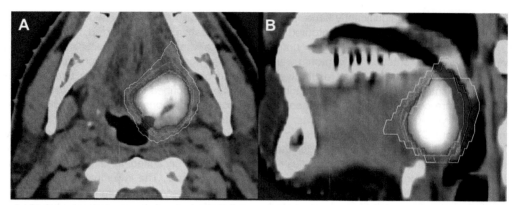

Fig. 4. PET-treatment planning CT fusion of an SCCA of the base of tongue shown in axial (*A*) and sagittal (*B*) planes. Automated segmentation and contouring of the primary tumor GTV based on PET SUV values using different segmentation techniques: absolute threshold SUV of 2.5 (*yellow*, 40 mL); absolute threshold SUV of 3.5 (*blue*, 29 mL); 40% of max SUV (*red*, 20 mL); and a gradient-based algorithm (*green*, 24 mL). Performed on MIM Vista software.

From the previously mentioned studies, it can be seen that the tumor volume can vary widely based on the segmentation methods used; however, the usefulness of this is limited unless it is in the context of pathology, which should be our gold standard. Burri and colleagues[41] showed that a threshold of 40% maximal SUV results in a good balance of not underestimating the tumor volume while improving on the visual and absolute SUV threshold methods. Newer gradient and adaptive threshold methods are promising but need to be validated by surgical specimens in other subsites.

TREATMENT OUTCOMES

The use of FDG-PET imaging results in differing target volumes, but it is important to understand the influence of PET imaging on patient outcomes. Does the use of PET imaging for radiation treatment planning improve patient outcomes? Unfortunately, there are no randomized trials comparing radiation treatment planning with or without the aid of FDG-PET imaging. Vernon and coinvestigators[48] reported on the outcomes of 42 patients treated with definitive radiation or chemoradiation with the aid of PET/CT imaging during radiation treatment planning. GTVs were contoured by a radiation oncologist and head-and-neck radiologist using an SUV threshold of 2.5. Eighty-six percent of patients had Stage III or IV disease and 83% of patients were treated with an IMRT technique, with the remaining treated with a 3-D-conformal technique. With a median follow-up of 32 months the 2-year overall survival and disease-free survival were 82.8% and 71%, respectively. Six patients, all with Stage III or IV

disease, experienced local failures with a 2-year locoregional control rate of 85.7%. They reported no correlation between local failure and maximum SUV of the primary tumor or nodes, but the analysis was limited by the small number of failures. Although only 86% of patients in the previously mentioned study were treated with IMRT, the results appear comparable with recent IMRT outcomes data. Yao and colleagues[49] reported a similar 2-year overall survival of 85% in patients treated with definitive or postoperative IMRT. Chao and coinvestigators[50] reported a 2-year actuarial rate of locoregional control of 85% in patients treated with definitive or postoperative IMRT. These data are similar to the outcomes of patients treated using PET-aided radiation treatment planning reported by Vernon and colleagues.[48] Further clinical trials with longer follow-up and incorporation of quality-of-life measurements are needed to determine the role of using FDG-PET in radiation treatment planning in patients with head and neck cancer.

NEW DIRECTIONS
Subvolume Delineation and Dose Escalation

Traditionally, the GTV, including the primary tumor and nodal volumes, are contoured in the treatment-planning CT with or without the aid of additional imaging modalities. An attempt is then made to prescribe a homogeneous dose to the PTVs. Most locoregional failures of head and neck cancer treated with IRMT occur in the high-dose regions,[51] suggesting that the radiation dose delivered may not be high enough and dose escalation is needed to better control the tumor. However, dose escalation to a large treatment volume may not ways be feasible and could cause significant toxicities. Tumors are not homogeneous structures and there are areas inside the tumor that may harbor more aggressive cancer cells. With the dose-painting capability of IMRT, a higher radiation dose can be delivered to tumor subvolumes that may be more radioresistant. FDG-avid regions in the tumor have been shown to be correlated with hypoxia that is associated with tumor radioresistance.[52,53] Higher pretreatment SUVs are associated with worse treatment outcomes, including worse disease-free survival and a decrease in local control.[54–56] Therefore, some groups have investigated the use of PET imaging to define a subvolume for dose escalation.

Schwartz and coinvestigators[21] studied theoretical IMRT models using PET-derived volumes compared with CT-derived volumes in 20 patients with head and neck cancer. Patients underwent contrasted CT scan and a PET scan while immobilized in the treatment position. CT and PET images were coregistered using a nonrigid algorithm. GTV-CT was derived from the CT data by radiologists who were blinded to the PET data, and GTV-PET was derived from the PET/CT data by nuclear medicine physicians using a visual method. Theoretical IMRT plans were constructed to deliver 66 Gy in 30 fractions to the PTV. They reported a significantly decreased mean contralateral parotid gland dose and mean larynx dose with PET/CT-directed IMRT as compared with CT-directed IMRT. In 5 patients, a theoretical dose-escalation plan was generated to deliver a boost to GTV-PET in a stepwise fashion with incremental 2.2-Gy fractions. Schwartz and coinvestigators[21] found that a mean dose of 74.9 Gy (range, 71.53–80.98 Gy) could be delivered without overdosing the adjacent critical structures.

Madani and colleagues[57] conducted a Phase I study of dose escalation to FDG-avid subvolumes. Patients underwent contrasted CT and PET scans of the head and neck immobilized in a mask. PET images were manually coregistered with CT data. CT-GTVs were delineated manually by investigators and PET-GTVs were delineated via an automated algorithm using a source-to-background method.[38] Dose escalation to the FDG-avid subvolumes was performed using an upfront, simultaneously integrated boost with IMRT. The IMRT was delivered in 2 phases. The first phase was delivered to a focal region defined by PET within the GTV with dose escalation at 2 levels: Group I (25 Gy in 10 fractions) and Group II (30 Gy in 10 fractions). Standard IMRT, consisting of 22 fractions of 2.16 Gy, was then given following the upfront boost with total doses delivered to PET subvolumes being 72.5 Gy and 77.5 Gy,

respectively. In Group II the investigators limited the volume that could receive the 3.0 Gy daily boost to 10 mL. If that volume was exceeded, the remaining volume received a 2.5-Gy daily boost. Macroscopic tumor on CT and enlarged lymph nodes were treated to 69 Gy and elective nodal areas were treated to 56 Gy. Toxicity was scored using National Cancer Institute Common Toxicity Criteria, version 2.0. A total of 41 patients were enrolled, 23 patients in Group I and 18 patients in Group II. Nine of 23 patients in Group I and 14 of 18 patients in Group II also received concurrent cisplatin-based chemotherapy. Thirty-nine patients completed treatment; only 2 of them required treatment breaks. Of the 2 patients requiring breaks, 1 was because of Grade 4 skin toxicity (5-day break) and the other was because of Grade 3 dysphagia requiring PEG placement (10-day break). Grade 2 or higher skin toxicity was the most common acute toxicity. Twenty-six percent of patients in Group I and 56% of patients in Group II required hospitalization at some point during treatment. One patient with locally advanced oropharyngeal cancer receiving concurrent chemotherapy died during treatment at 53 Gy as a result of sepsis, which halted further enrollment as per protocol. No patients experienced any late Grade 4 toxicities. Fibrosis and dysphagia were the most common late toxicities with Grades 1 to 3 dysphagia occurring in 50% and 90% of patients in Groups I and II, respectively. A complete tumor response was seen in 85.7% of Group I and 81.2% of Group II patients. The actuarial overall survival at 1 year was 82% in Group I and 54% in Group II ($P = .06$). The patients in Group II tended to have larger GTVs and had more laryngeal and pharyngeal tumors. Locoregional control at 1 year was 85% and 87% respectively. Seven patients had a local recurrence. More than half (4/7) of local recurrences occurred inside the PET-GTV–defined area that received the dose escalation, suggesting that FDG-PET could be used to detect relapse-prone regions. This study highlights the feasibility of dose escalation to a PET-defined subvolume. The investigators are planning a randomized phase II trial comparing the dose prescription at dose level II with standard IMRT.

Adaptive Radiation Therapy

During the course of radiotherapy, a patient can have significant physical/anatomic changes owing to tumor response that requires a second CT simulation and replanning to ensure the tumor is being dosed appropriately. Changes also occur in the FDG uptake of the tumor during the course of radiotherapy, and some investigators have explored adaptive radiotherapy and planning techniques to alter the plan based on PET imaging.

Moule and coinvestigators[58] studied functional volumes in 10 patients and how they changed on PET/CT during therapy. PET/CT scans were obtained pretreatment and at the following dose time points: 8 to 18 Gy, 36 to 50 Gy, and 66 Gy. Volumes were defined using an adaptive iterative algorithm weighted according to the mean SUV. Using this technique to define volumes, the group noted no significant reduction in the primary target volumes during radiotherapy. However, the nodal target volumes were noted to decrease during treatment. The maximum SUV of both the primary and nodal targets were also noted to decrease during treatment but because of difficulties with the algorithm distinguishing the SUV of the tumor from the background activity, the investigators did not advocate for using PET during treatment to redefine tumor volumes.

Hentschel and colleagues[59] also explored how PET-defined volumes changed during radiotherapy treatment. GTVs from PET were defined by a source-to-background algorithm for pretreatment scans and at 3 time points during treatment. They noted a decrease in the median SUVmax during therapy; however, the median GTV-PET volume increased during the course of therapy. The investigators concluded that this was because of an increase in inflammation during the radiation course and that it was not possible to create an adaptive plan based on PET changes during therapy using this technique.

Duprez and coworkers[60] studied the feasibility of treating patients with an adaptive technique using dose painting by numbers (DPBN) in a Phase I trial. Two dose levels were explored, 80.5 Gy and 85.9 Gy, to the primary tumor using dose painting with IMRT based on PET-voxel intensity to dose escalate an intratumoral volume. This adaptive technique based on PET was performed for fractions 1 to 10 and another adaptive plan from a pertreatment PET was delivered for fractions 11 to 20, followed by a conventional (non–dose painted) IMRT plan. The investigators delineated the PET target volume by a threshold technique of 50% of SUVmax. All 21 patients on the trial completed therapy without a break and no Grade 4 toxicities were encountered. The investigators noted that the GTV based on the adaptive PET decreased by 41%. Tumor control rates were not reported. The investigators concluded that DPBN using an adaptive plan based on pretreatment and pertreatment PET scan was feasible and tolerated.

Investigators report changes in PET SUVmax values during treatment, but delineation of the tumor volume is still challenging at the border because of the increasing inflammatory response during a course of radiotherapy. Adaptive treatment plans based on PET could lead to underdosing the tumor, and these techniques should be used only in the context of clinical trials.

Other Tracers

FDG is the most frequently used radiopharmaceutical for PET imaging. It is widely available and has a clinically practical half-life of 110 minutes. However, FDG has limitations, which include normal physiologic uptake in brain, kidney, active muscle, lymphoid tissues, brown fat, and inflamed tissues. In the head and neck region, lymphoid tissues in the tonsils and base of tongue often have increased FDG uptake, which may lead to an overestimation of the tumor volume based on FDG uptake. An ideal replacement would be more specific for malignancy than FDG, while being widely available and having an acceptable half-life.

Methionine was been shown to reflect increased amino acid transport and protein synthesis in malignant tissue. Geets and colleagues[61] compared GTVs derived from 11C-methionine-PET (MET-PET) with those derived from CT and FDG PET. GTVs from PET images were delineated using an adaptive threshold method that took into account the source-to-background ratio. With 21 patients, they reported no significant difference between the volumes delineated from CT alone versus MET-PET in laryngeal and oropharyngeal tumors. However, as noted in other studies, FDG PET volumes were significantly smaller when compared with CT alone. The investigators suggested that the larger MET-PET volumes were likely because of high physiologic uptake in the submandibular glands, mucosa, and bone marrow.

Several investigators have performed feasibility studies using hypoxic tracers to define subvolumes for dose escalation to the hypoxic component of the tumor. Because hypoxia is related to radioresistance, and the hypoxic area in the tumor may contain more aggressive and radioresistant cancer cells, higher dose to the hypoxic volume might lead to improved local control. Several hypoxia radiotracers have been developed. Theoretically, these tracers are bioreductive molecules that accept an election in the reductive/hypoxic environment of a tumor with the resultant reduced molecule being unable to leave the malignant cell. Chao and colleagues[62] studied the hypoxia tracer [60-Cu]Cu (II)-diacetylbis (N4-methylthiosemicarbazone) (Cu-ATSM). A theoretical IMRT dose escalation plan was constructed using a hypoxia ubvolume defined by Cu-ATSM-PET in a patient with a tonsil/base of tongue cancer. A threshold twice the background uptake in neck muscle as used to define the hypoxic volume. The theoretical plan was able to successfully deliver D Gy in 35 fractions to the subvolume while maintaining normal structure constraints. Grosu and colleagues[63] studied the hypoxia tracer [18F] fluoroazomycin-arabinoside (FAZA) in 18 patients with head and neck cancer. GTVs delineated on CT were compared with subvolumes corresponding to FAZA-PET imaging using an SUV larger than 50% of the mean SUV in neck muscle as the delineation method. Theoretical IMRT plans were constructed to provide a boost to total dose of 80.5 Gy to the hypoxic subvolumes. They were able to delineate a hypoxic subvolume for the primary tumor in 15 of 18 patients. The FAZA-GTV for the primary tumor failed to correlate significantly with the CT-GTV and represented only a median of 10.8% of the CT-GTV (range 0.7%–52.0%). For the lymph nodes, hypoxic subvolumes were able to be delineated in only 10 of 16 patients. In contrast to the primary tumors, the nodal hypoxic subvolumes correlated significantly with the nodal CT-GTVs. Grosu and colleagues[63] reported that in 2% of patients, the hypoxic subvolumes were not contiguous as would be expected. This could have led to the lack of correlation between GTV-FAZA and GTV-CT in the primary tumor. They also showed that the theoretical IMRT plan giving 0.5 Gy to the hypoxic subvolume did not increase radiation dose to the critical structures. Lee and colleagues[64] studied the feasibility of dose escalation to subvolumes detected by hypoxia tracer [18F] fluoromisonidazole (FMISO). Theoretical IMRT plans were designed for 10 patients giving 0 Gy to the FDG-PET/CT GTV and a boost to a total dose of 84 Gy to the hypoxic subvolumes inside the GTV as defined by FMISO-PET. Lee and colleagues[64] showed that this can be achieved in all 10 patients without exceeding the normal tissue tolerances. Other plans were explored to boost the hypoxic subvolume to 105 Gy in 2 patients, which was successful in 1 patient with a relatively small hypoxia subvolume. Lin and colleagues[65] in the same group also performed a feasibility study for dose escalation using FMISO-PET and evaluated the reproducibility of the FMISO-PET scan by obtaining 2 scans separated by 3 days before radiotherapy. When comparing the serial FMISO-PET scans, they found that the hypoxic volume had significantly changed in 4 of 7 patients, which could have compromised the planned boost dose. The inconsistency in the hypoxic volume between 2 scans can be attributed to a variety of causes, such as

technical issues, but tumor hypoxia is not a static process and can change over time, especially after treatment when reoxygenation occurs. Further studies are necessary for the implication for subvolume delineation using hypoxia tracers.

These studies demonstrate the feasibility of designing subvolumes based on radiopharmaceuticals other than FDG. However, further clinical trials are necessary to determine if dose escalation to the hypoxic regions could lead to improved local control of the disease.

SUMMARY

FDG-PET imaging is being used more frequently by radiation oncologists for radiation treatment planning. PET is a powerful tool that provides metabolic/biologic data that can aid the oncologist in staging, treatment planning, and patient management. New gradient and adaptive threshold algorithms appear promising with regard to segmentation and may reduce variability among radiation oncologists. We may find that the optimal segmentation method may vary according to subsite (eg, glottis, base of tongue) and tumor biology, such as grade or HPV status. Adaptive planning using PET scans during treatment is under investigation, and studies in dose escalation to PET volumes will hopefully lead to improved local control of tumor although randomized trials comparing dose escalation to conventional IMRT are needed. Finally, advances in PET and CT technology will hopefully lead to continued improvements in resolution and new radiotracers will enable us to better refine the specific metabolic process in tumors for target delineation.

REFERENCES

1. Siegel R, Naishadham D, Jemal A. Cancer statistics, 2012. CA. Cancer J Clin 2012;62:10–29.
2. Adelstein DL, Li Y, Adams GL, et al. An intergroup phase III comparison of standard radiation and two schedules of concurrent chemoradiotherapy in patients with unresectable squamous cell head and neck cancer. J Clin Oncol 2003;21:92–8.
3. Forastiere AA, Goepfert H, Maor M, et al. Concurrent chemotherapy and radiotherapy for organ preservation in advanced laryngeal cancer. N Engl J Med 2003;329:2091–8.
4. Al-Sarraf M, LeBlanc M, Giri PG, et al. Chemoradiotherapy versus radiotherapy in patients with advanced nasopharyngeal cancer: phase III randomized Intergroup study 0099. J Clin Oncol 1998;16: 1310–7.
5. Cooper JS, Pajak TF, Forastiere AA, et al. Postoperative concurrent radiotherapy and chemotherapy for

high-risk squamous-cell carcinoma of the head and neck. N Engl J Med 2004;350:1937–44.

6. Bernier J, Domenge C, Ozsahim M, et al. Postoperative irradiation with or without concomitant chemotherapy for locally advanced head and neck cancer. N Engl J Med 2004;350:1945–52.

7. Mell L, Mehrotra A, Mundt A. Intensity-modulated radiation therapy use in the US, 2004. Cancer 2005;104:1296–303.

8. Lee N, Puri D, Blanco A, et al. Intensity-modulated radiation therapy in head and neck cancers: an update. Head Neck 2007;29:387–400.

9. Gregoire V, De Neve W, Eisbruch A, et al. Intensity-modulated radiation therapy for head and neck carcinoma. Oncologist 2007;12:555–64.

10. Chao KS, Deasy J, Markman J, et al. A prospective study of salivary function sparing in patients with head-and-neck cancers receiving intensity-modulated or three-dimensional radiation therapy: initial results. Int J Radiat Oncol Biol Phys 2001;49:907–16.

11. Lin A, Kim HM, Terrell J, et al. Quality of life after parotid-sparing IMRT for head-and-neck cancer: a prospective longitudinal study. Int J Radiat Oncol Biol Phys 2003;57:61–70.

12. Yao M, Karnell LH, Funk GF, et al. Health-related quality-of-life outcomes following IMRT versus conventional radiotherapy for oropharyngeal squamous cell carcinoma. Int J Radiat Oncol Biol Phys 2007;69:1354–60.

13. Roh J, Yeo N, Kim JS, et al. Utility of 2-[18F] fluoro-2-deoxy-D-glucose positron emission tomography and positron emission tomography/computed tomography imaging in the preoperative staging of head and neck squamous cell carcinoma. Oral Oncol 2007;43:887–93.

14. Ng S, Yen T, Liao C, et al. 18F-FDG PET and CT/MRI in oral cavity squamous cell carcinoma: a prospective study of 124 patients with histologic correlation. J Nucl Med 2005;46:1136–43.

15. Al-Ibraheem A, Buck A, Krause BJ, et al. Clinical applications of FDG PET and PET/CT in head and neck cancer. J Oncol 2009;2009:208725.

16. McCollum AD, Burrell S, Haddad R, et al. Positron emission tomography with 18F-fluorodeoxyglucose to predict pathologic response after induction chemotherapy and definitive chemoradiotherapy in head and neck cancer. Head Neck 2004;26:890–6.

17. Yen R, Chen TH, Ting L, et al. Early restaging whole-body 18F-FDG PET during induction chemotherapy predicts clinical outcome in patients with locoregionally advanced nasopharyngeal carcinoma. Eur J Nucl Med Mol Imaging 2005;32:1152–9.

18. Yao M, Smith R, Hoffman H, et al. Clinical significance of postradiotherapy 18F-fluorodeoxyglucose positron emission tomography imaging in management of head-and-neck cancer—a long term outcome report. Int J Radiat Oncol Biol Phys 200 74:9–14.

19. Gupta T, Master Z, Kannan S, et al. Diagnost performance of post-treatment FDG PET or FD PET/CT imaging in head and neck cancer: a sy temic review and meta-analysis. Eur J Nucl Me Mol Imaging 2011;38:2083–95.

20. Simpson DR, Lawson JD, Nath SK, et al. Utilization advanced imaging technologies for target delinea tion in radiation oncology. J Am Coll Radiol 2009; 876–83.

21. Schwartz D, Ford EC, Rajendran J, et al. FDG-PE CT-guided intensity modulated head and neck radi therapy: a pilot investigation. Head Neck 2005;2 478–87.

22. Mattes D, Haynor D, Vesselle H, et al. PET-CT imag registration in the chest using free-form deforma tions. IEEE Trans Med Imaging 2003;22:120–8.

23. Vogel WV, Schinagl DA, Van Dalen JA, et al. Va dated image fusion of dedicated PET and CT f external beam radiation and therapy in the hea and neck area. Q J Nucl Med Mol Imaging 200 52:74–83.

24. Ireland R, Dyker K, Barber D, et al. Nonrigid imag registration for head and neck cancer radiotherap treatment planning with PET/CT. Int J Radiat Onc Biol Phys 2007;68:952–7.

25. Hwang AB, Bacharach SL, Yom SS, et al. Can pos tron emission tomography (PET) or PET/Compute Tomography (CT) acquired in a nontreatment pos tion be accurately registered to a head-and-nec radiotherapy planning CT? Int J Radiat Oncol Bi Phys 2009;73:578–84.

26. Park SB, Rhee FC, Monroe JI, et al. Spatial weighte mutual information for image registration in imag guided radiation therapy. Med Phys 2008;35:2855

27. Ciernik IF, Dizendorf E, Baumert BG, et al. Radiatio treatment planning with an integrated positron emis sion and computer tomography (PET/CT): a feas bility study. Int J Radiat Oncol Biol Phys 2003;5 853–63.

28. Paulino AC, Koshy M, Howell R, et al. Comparison c CT- and FDG-PET-defined gross tumor volume i intensity-modulated radiotherapy for head-and-nec cancer. Int J Radiat Oncol Biol Phys 2005;61:1385–9

29. Deantonio L, Beldì D, Gambaro G, et al. FDG-PE CT imaging for staging and radiotherapy treatmer planning of head and neck carcinoma. Radiat Onc 2008;3:29.

30. Guido A, Fuccio L, Rombi B, et al. Combined 18F FDG-PET/CT imaging in radiotherapy target delinea tion for head-and-neck cancer. Int J Radiat Onc Biol Phys 2009;73:759–63.

31. Scarfone C, Lavely WC, Cmelak AJ, et al. Prospec tive feasibility trial of radiotherapy target definitio for head and neck cancer using 3-dimension PET and CT imaging. J Nucl Med 2004;45:543–52.

2. El-Bassiouni M, Ciernik IF, Davis JB, et al. [18FDG] PET-CT-based intensity-modulated radiotherapy treatment planning of head and neck cancer. Int J Radiat Oncol Biol Phys 2007;69:286–93.

3. Henriques de Figueiredo B, Barret O, Demeaux H, et al. Comparison between CT- and FDG-PET-defined target volumes for radiotherapy planning in head-and-neck cancers. Radiother Oncol 2009;93: 479–82.

4. Wang D, Schultz CJ, Jursinic PA, et al. Initial experience of FDG-PET/CT guided IMRT of head-and-neck carcinoma. Int J Radiat Oncol Biol Phys 2006;65:143–51.

5. Heron DE, Andrade RS, Flickinger J, et al. Hybrid PET-CT simulation for radiation treatment planning in head-and-neck cancers: a brief technical report. Int J Radiat Oncol Biol Phys 2004;60:1419–24.

6. Schinagl DA, Vogel WV, Hoffmann AL, et al. Comparison of five segmentation tools for 18F-fluoro-deoxy-glucose-positron emission tomography-based target volume definition in head and neck cancer. Int J Radiat Oncol Biol Phys 2007;69:1282–9.

7. Greco C, Nehmeh SA, Schöder H, et al. Evaluation of different methods of 18F-FDG-PET target volume delineation in the radiotherapy of head and neck cancer. Am J Clin Oncol 2008;31:439–45.

8. Daisne J, Sibomana M, Bol A, et al. Tri-dimensional automatic segmentation of PET volumes based on measured source-to-background ratios: influence of reconstruction algorithms. Radiother Oncol 2003; 69:247–50.

9. Adams R, Bischof L. Seeded region growing. IEEE Trans Pattern Anal Mach Intell 1994;16:641–7.

40. Hsu PK, Huang HC, Hsieh CC, et al. Effect of formalin fixation on tumor size determination in stage I non-small cell lung cancer. Ann Thorac Surg 2007; 84:1825–9.

41. Burri RJ, Rangaswamy B, Kostakoglu L, et al. Correlation of positron emission tomography standard uptake value and pathologic specimen size in cancer of the head and neck. Int J Radiat Oncol Biol Phys 2008;71:682–8.

42. Daisne JF, Duprez T, Weynand B, et al. Tumor volume in pharyngolaryngeal squamous cell carcinoma: comparison at CT, MR imaging, and FDG PET and validation with surgical specimen. Radiology 2004;233:93–100.

43. Seitz O, Chambron-Pinho N, Middendorp M, et al. 18F-Fluorodeoxyglucose-PET/CT to evaluate tumor, nodal disease, and gross tumor volume of oropharyngeal and oral cavity cancer: comparison with MR imaging and validation with surgical specimen. Neuroradiology 2009;51:677–86.

44. Geets X, Lee JA, Bol A, et al. A gradient-based method for segmenting FDG-PET images: methodology and validation. Eur J Nucl Med Mol Imaging 2007;34:1427–38.

45. Murphy JD, Chisholm KM, Daly ME, et al. Correlation between metabolic tumor volume and pathologic tumor volume in squamous cell carcinoma of the oral cavity. Radiother Oncol 2011;101:356–61.

46. Zaidi H, Abdoli M, Fuentes CL, et al. Comparative methods for PET image segmentation in pharyngo-laryngeal squamous cell carcinoma. Eur J Nucl Med Mol Imaging 2012;39:881–91.

47. Zaidi H, El Naqa I. PET-guided delineation of radiation therapy treatment volumes: a survey of image segmentation techniques. Eur J Nucl Med Mol Imaging 2010;37:1935–7.

48. Vernon MR, Maheshwari M, Schultz CJ, et al. Clinical outcomes of patients receiving integrated PET/CT-guided radiotherapy for head and neck carcinoma. Int J Radiat Oncol Biol Phys 2008;70:678–84.

49. Yao M, Dornfeld KJ, Buatti JM, et al. Intensity-modulated radiation treatment for head-and-neck squamous cell carcinoma—the University of Iowa experience. Int J Radiat Oncol Biol Phys 2005;63:410–21.

50. Chao KS, Ozyigit G, Tran BN, et al. Patterns of failure in patients receiving definitive and postoperative IMRT for head-and-neck cancer. Int J Radiat Oncol Biol Phys 2003;55:312–21.

51. Dawson LA, Anzai Y, Marsh L, et al. Patterns of local-regional recurrence following parotid-sparing conformal and segmental intensity-modulated radiotherapy for head and neck cancer. Int J Radiat Oncol Biol Phys 2000;46:1117–26.

52. Mees G, Dierckx R, Vangestel C, et al. Molecular imaging of hypoxia with radiolabelled agents. Eur J Nucl Med Mol Imaging 2009;36:1674–86.

53. Pugachev A, Ruan S, Carlin S, et al. Dependence of FDG uptake on tumor microenvironment. Int J Radiat Oncol Biol Phys 2005;62:545–53.

54. Allal AS, Slosman DO, Kebdani T, et al. Prediction of outcome in head-and-neck cancer patients using the standardized uptake value of 2-[18F]fluoro-2-deoxy-D-glucose. Int J Radiat Oncol Biol Phys 2004; 59:1295–300.

55. Machtay M, Natwa M, Andrel J, et al. Pretreatment FDG-PET standardized uptake value as a prognostic factor for outcome in head and neck cancer. Head Neck 2009;31:195–201.

56. Yao M, Lu M, Savvides P, et al. The prognostic significance of pretreatment SUV in head-and-neck squamous cell carcinoma treated with IMRT. Int J Radiat Oncol Biol Phys 2009;75:S17.

57. Madani I, Duthoy W, Derie C, et al. Positron emission tomography-guided, focal-dose escalation using intensity-modulated radiotherapy for head and neck cancer. Int J Radiat Oncol Biol Phys 2007;68:126–35.

58. Moule RN, Kayani I, Prior T, et al. Adaptive FDG positron emission tomography/computed tomography-based target volume delineation in radiotherapy planning of head and neck cancer. Clinical Onc 2011;23:364–71.

59. Hentschel M, Appold S, Schreiber A, et al. Serial FDG-PET on patients with head and neck cancer: implications for radiation therapy. Int J Radiat Biol 2009;85:796–804.

60. Duprez F, De Neve W, De Gersem W, et al. Adaptive dose painting by numbers for head-and-neck cancer. Int J Radiat Oncol Biol Phys 2011;80:1045–55.

61. Geets X, Daisne JF, Gregoire V, et al. Role of 11-C-methionine positron emission tomography for the delineation of the tumor volume in pharyngo-laryngeal squamous cell carcinoma: comparison with FDG-PET and CT. Radiother Oncol 2004;71:267–73.

62. Chao KS, Bosch WR, Mutic S, et al. A novel approach to overcome hypoxic tumor resistance: Cu-ATSM-guided intensity-modulated radiation therapy. Int J Radiat Oncol Biol Phys 2001;49:1171–82.

63. Grosu AL, Souvatzoglou M, Röper B, et al. Hypoxia imaging with FAZA-PET and theoretical considerations with regard to dose painting for individualization of radiotherapy in patients with head and neck cancer. Int J Radiat Oncol Biol Phys 2007;6 541–51.

64. Lee N, Mechalakos JG, Nehmeh S, et al. Fluorine-18 labeled fluoromisonidazole positron emission and computed tomography-guided intensity-modulated radiotherapy for head-and-neck cancer: a feasibility study. Int J Radiat Oncol Biol Phys 2008;70:2–13.

65. Lin Z, Mechalakos JG, Nehmeh S, et al. The influence of changes in tumor hypoxia on dose-painting treatment planes based on ^{18}F-FMISO positron emission tomography. Int J Radiat Oncol Biol Phys 2008;7 1219–28.

PET in Decision Making for Neck Dissection After Radiation Treatment

Gerard Adams, BSc(Hons), MBChB, MRCP, FRCR, FRANZCR[a],
Sandro V. Porceddu, MBBS(Hons), FRANZCR, MD[a,b],*

KEYWORDS

- PET-CT • Head & neck squamous cell carcinoma (HNSCC) • Node positive (N+) • Radiotherapy
- Chemoradiotherapy • Neck dissection

KEY POINTS

- Isolated nodal relapse is uncommon after chemoradiation for head and neck squamous cell carcinoma when there has been a complete response at the primary site.
- Neck dissection after chemoradiation can result in substantial long-term toxicity and impaired quality of life.
- A PET-directed policy is safe and cost-effective in selecting those who can be spared neck dissection while allowing surgery to those who may benefit.

INTRODUCTION

Organ-preserving definitive therapy with chemoradiation for locally advanced head and neck squamous cell carcinoma (HNSCC) is now well established.[1] Historically, there have been controversies about the requirement for additional surgical intervention in the neck. This controversy is especially true in patients with positive neck nodes (N+) after a complete response at the primary site. Options include an up-front neck dissection before radiotherapy, a planned neck dissection after treatment, or a more selective approach using posttreatment assessment of response (ranging from simple clinical examination to more sophisticated anatomic and functional imaging) to select patients who may be safely spared neck dissection.[2] These differing approaches reflect the competing desires to maximize the chance of locoregional control while minimizing the burden of treatment-related toxicity in survivors. Over the last 20 years, the consensus of opinion has evolved toward a more selective approach to choosing patients for neck dissection. There are several factors that have contributed to this change.

Improvements in the Effectiveness of Modern Treatments

Developments, such as concurrent chemoradiation,[3] hyperfractionated,[4] and/or accelerated radiotherapy,[4–6] coupled with improvements in delivering treatment, including 3-dimensional conformal and intensity-modulated radiotherapy, mean that locoregional control rates are likely to be higher in the modern era than earlier reports suggest.

The Changing Biology of HNSCC

With decreasing rates of smoking, a larger proportion of HNSCCs (particularly of the oropharynx) are related to the human papilloma virus (HPV). These

Disclosures: None.
a Division of Cancer Services, Department of Radiation Oncology, Princess Alexandra Hospital, 199 Ipswich Road, Queensland 4102, Australia; b Faculty of Health Sciences, School of Medicine, University of Queensland, St Lucia, Brisbane, Queensland 4072, Australia
* Corresponding author.
E-mail address: Sandro_Porceddu@health.qld.gov.au

PET Clin 7 (2012) 411–423
http://dx.doi.org/10.1016/j.cpet.2012.06.004

tumors are more likely to present with enlarged lymph nodes but also seem to have a significantly better prognosis regardless of the treatment modality.[7] Therefore, this brings into question any policy that dictates neck dissection following a complete response at the primary site that is based on the nodal stage alone.

The Impact of Complications of Multimodality Treatment

Complications from planned neck dissection after chemoradiation occur at rates of around 12% for severe (grade 3 or 4) and 35% for minor (grade 1 or 2) complications.[8] Those who undergo neck dissection after chemoradiation also have significantly higher rates of severe long-term toxicities[9] and pain affecting their quality of life.[10]

Indeed, the very low rate of isolated neck failure in those patients who demonstrate a complete response at both the primary and nodal sites after chemoradiation and who do not undergo a neck dissection,[11] coupled with the significant burden of additional toxicity that a neck dissection places on long-term survivors, means that we are duty bound to find effective strategies to identify those patients who can avoid unnecessary neck dissection while maintaining high locoregional control rates.

To date, there is no firm consensus as to what that strategy should be. Challenges include identifying an appropriate outcome measure (pathologic node positivity or isolated nodal relapse), identifying the correct timing of assessment so as not to miss the window of opportunity in those who require intervention, and identifying the most efficient and cost-effective combination of tools to use.

The focus of this article is to discuss the evidence for and the controversies surrounding the use of PET in treatment decisions after definitive chemoradiation for HNSCC. The discussion almost exclusively surrounds the use of [18]fluorodeoxyglucose-PET (FDG-PET) in N+ disease. The utility of FDG-PET in the initial evaluation of the neck is addressed in the chapter by Andrew Quon while the use of tracers other than FDG is discussed in the chapter by Yusuf Menda, Nancy Lee and Tony J Wang.

Planned Neck Dissection

Protocols for planned neck dissection in combination with radiotherapy were developed in the 1970s, such as those from the MD Anderson Cancer Center.[12] However, evidence supporting this approach is scant. Only one randomized trial evaluating the effectiveness of planned neck dissection in the context of definitive chemoradiation exists.[13] In this small trial of 54 patients who

were likely treated with suboptimal doses of radiation (doses equivalent to 60 or 65 Gy over 6 or weeks), there were improvements in disease-free survival at both 2 years (52% vs 26%) and 5 year (29% vs 0%) favoring the group undergoing a planned neck dissection before chemoradiation

Retrospective studies suggest that in N2 and N disease, a planned neck dissection following radio therapy results in improvements in local neck control[14] and possibly causes specific survival. Other researchers have looked at the rates of residual cancer cells in neck dissection specimen after definitive chemoradiation. They reveal histologically positive rates as high as 40% in case adjudged to have a complete clinical response.[16–18] This finding, along with concerns that nodal disease may somehow be more radioresistant than primary disease,[19] and the extreme poor survival rates when neck relapse is treated with salvage neck dissection[20,21] support the role of planned neck dissection for all.

Selective Approach to Neck Dissection

A neck dissection for all (either up-front, before radiation, or planned to take place after the completion of treatment) means that all patients are subjected to the risks and complications of neck surgery regardless of the response to treatment. Indeed, the studies of Lavertu and Stenson[17,18] showed that all patients with N1 disease and complete response to chemoradiation had negative pathologic specimens and a very low risk of subsequent recurrence.

In contrast to the planned neck dissection approach outlined earlier, primarily from work done at the University of Florida, protocols evolved to omitting neck dissection for solitary nodes less than 3 cm (N1)[22] and then to a policy of neck dissection only for those individuals who fail to demonstrate a complete clinical and radiologic response to treatment, regardless of the N stage.[2] However, these protocols are not universally accepted. Some groups still advocate an up-front planned neck dissection for all patients with N or N3 diseases[24] or high-risk primary sites, such as pyriform sinus, regardless of the nodal stage[2] and regardless of the clinical response.

How to Assess Clinical Response to Treatment

Frequent routine physical examination by an experienced physician is vitally important in the follow up of patients after chemoradiation. However because of the physical changes within the neck it is unlikely to be sufficient on its own to detect low-volume residual or recurrent disease in asymptomatic patients who have completed treatment.[2]

omputerized Tomography Scan

aditionally, because of the limitations of physical xaminations, the definition of complete response ombines both negative findings on physical xamination and the absence of nodes on aging, usually computed tomography (CT).

In a retrospective series that correlated the findgs of CT scans performed shortly after radioerapy with pathologic findings from a planned eck dissection, Ojiri and colleagues[27] were able identify a series of factors that were highly redictive of negative pathologic findings. These ctors were

- Lymph node size of 5 mm or less
- The absence of nodal internal focal deficits
- No evidence of extracapsular extension

From 113 neck dissections, 37 (33%) were posive for residual disease. Only 1 out of 29 cases ith a negative CT finding resulted in positive stopathology (negative predictive value [NPV] f 97%). These findings led to the change in policy t the University of Florida allowing for the elimina-on of routine neck dissection in those with a radio-gic complete response after treatment.[23]

However, following these criteria would still ean that 42% (48 out of 113) of patients are sub-cted to the potential complications of neck issection with no apparent benefit because there ill be no residual pathologic cells. In addition, only 3% (36 out of 84) of neck dissections performed ould have a positive histopathology—a finding at alone does not necessarily indicate viable isease.

There is an increasing body of clinical evidence o support the notion that a negative CT scan per-ormed shortly after completion of treatment can elp define complete response and safely elimi-ate the need for a planned neck dissection. In n analysis from a randomized trial by the Trans asman Radiation Oncology Group (TROG 98–2)[11] whereby patients with N2 or N3 disease but ith a complete clinical and radiological response t the primary and nodal sites were followed by bservation of the neck rather than planned neck issection, no patients suffered an isolated nodal elapse.

More recently, Thariat and colleagues,[28] from the 1D Anderson Cancer Center, have reported their nalysis of 880 patients with locally advanced carci-omas of the oropharynx, larynx, or hypopharynx eated with radiation with or without chemotherapy etween 1994 and 2004 and followed for a median f 51 months. Throughout the time period of this tudy, their policy was to observe those patients ith a complete clinical and radiological response

at the nodal site regardless of the initial nodal status. This policy was from their previous study from 1996[29] in which 62 patients with N+ disease with oropharyngeal cancer and a complete radiological response had an isolated neck failure rate of less than 5% after observation.

In the larger study, a complete response was found in 377 (43%) patients based on a physical examination and CT performed 4 to 8 weeks after treatment. CT definition of complete response was similar to that previously described by Ojiri.[27] Of these, 377 365 (97%) were observed without planned neck dissection. Only 1 of the 12 complete responders who underwent a planned neck dissection had viable tumor cells in the specimen. A total of 26 failures in the neck developed in the 365 observed patients (7%).

However, of the 268 patients with incomplete nodal response who underwent neck dissection, a viable tumor was found in only 80 (30%). The 5-year regional control rates were similar for those undergoing observation after complete response (92%) and those undergoing neck dissection after a less-than-complete response (90%); overall, the rate of isolated neck failure was 4%.

In summary, when using CT criteria, it is safe to omit a planned neck dissection in those patients who have a clinical and radiological complete response to treatment based on an assessment taking place 4 to 8 weeks after the completion of therapy because the rate of isolated nodal relapse is very low. However, following such a policy would still result in more than half of the patients under-going neck dissection and up to 70% of these specimens would be negative for viable cells. Therefore, a policy directed by a single CT on completion of treatment is an improvement on a policy dictated on pretreatment nodal stage but still results in substantial overtreatment of the neck.

An alternative CT-based approach may involve patients with borderline residual lymph nodes being observed with serial imaging over time. If these continue to regress, it may be safe to omit neck dissection. This policy would spare some patients from an unnecessary neck dissection but to the detriment of others whereby the nodes do not shrink and the required neck dissection will be tech-nically more challenging because of fibrosis.

Ultrasound-Guided Cytology

Ultrasound-guided fine-needle aspiration cytology is highly accurate in the pretreatment assessment of the neck. However, its usefulness after radio-therapy is somewhat reduced. In a study by van der Putten and colleagues,[30] 46 patients undergoing neck dissection for residual or recurrent disease after definitive chemoradiation underwent fine-needle aspiration of suspicious lymph nodes before surgery. Thirty cytology samples were positive but only 12 (40%) ultimately contained viable tumor. Also, 3 of the 16 (19%) of the negative cytology samples were taken from necks that were ultimately shown to have residual tumor. Therefore, it was concluded that ultrasound-guided fine-needle aspiration cytology cannot accurately provide additional information when forming management plans for those who do not show a complete response at the neck nodes following chemoradiation.

Magnetic Resonance Imaging

Although there is evidence that CT and magnetic resonance (MR) imaging are equivalent in the pre-therapy staging of neck nodes,[31] there is little evidence evaluating MR imaging in the posttreatment setting.

FDG-PET

The well-established role of functional imaging with FDG-PET in the staging are discussed elsewhere in this issue by Andrew Quon and initial treatment of HNSCC are discussed elsewhere in this issue by Charles Wood and Min Yao. However, the main focus of this article is its role in the management of the neck after definitive chemoradiation.

As discussed earlier, the value of CT is in its high NPV, which allows neck dissection to be omitted in those who fulfill the radiological criteria for complete response. However, the presence of residual structural abnormalities in a significant proportion of patients means that if these criteria are universally applied, then ultimately a large proportion of patients will still undergo a neck dissection with high rates of pathologically negative samples.[28]

When PET is performed alone, the limited spatial resolution, lack of anatomic landmarks, and normal physiologic uptake of some structures may limit the interpretation of results, especially in the complex area of the head and neck.[32] However, the combination of metabolic and anatomic imaging with combined PET-CT scan is undoubtedly superior to CT alone or MR imaging in accurately identifying disease in the pretreatment setting.[33]

There has been a considerable research focus in assessing the use of PET to better select patients for neck dissection. This focus initially began with retrospective studies[34–39] suggesting that the addition of FEG-PET can maintain the high NPV but improve on the poor positive predictive value (PPV) of CT with the potential to ultimately improve the accuracy of assessment and reduce the number of neck dissections required.

Yao and colleagues[35] retrospectively reviewe 53 patients, with 70 heminecks to evaluate, wh underwent CT and PET 2 to 6 months after cheme radiation for N+ HNSCC. There was residual lymph adenopathy in 28 heminecks, 7 of which we positive on PET. Ultimately, 3 out of 7 PET positi heminecks were found to contain patholog evidence of residual tumor. Just as importantly, a 21 with residual lymph nodes on CT but that wee PET negative had no evidence of residual disea based on negative pathologic findings (4) or r evidence of neck relapse on subsequent follow-u (17). The NPV of PET was 100% and the PPV wa 42%. However, the retrospective nature of th and other studies along with the nonconsiste approach to management of the neck with regal to surgery meant that, although promising, a PE directed policy required further evaluation before could be adopted as the standard practice.

This finding has lead to 3 prospectiv cohorts[40–42] and 1 randomized trial[43] that hav been set up to address the question of the utili of PET in management decisions in the posttrea ment neck. To date, 2 of the cohorts have bee reported in full with the other appearing in abstra only. **Table 1** summarizes the studies and their ke findings as well as those from the large CT-base series published by Thariat and colleagues[28] tha was discussed previously.

The UK National Cancer Research Counci sponsored PET-NECK phase 3 trial is current active. As of April 2012, it had recruited 83% the 560-patient target and is expected to complet recruitment in September 2012.

MD Anderson Study

In the study by Moeller and colleagues,[40] 10 consecutive patients with locally advanced HNSC due to be treated with chemoradiation wer screened. Nine were ineligible and 6 censore because of the development of distant relaps before locoregional recurrence, leaving a total 92 for analysis. The aim of this study was to evaluat the utility of PET as a global tool to assess respons and not to direct the management of the nec specifically.

Patient characteristics, including the site and and N stage, were similar to the Brisbane an Canadian studies. Although mention is made assaying for HPV status, no results are reportec In a similar way to the other studies, CT and PE scans were performed after treatment (in thi case, with a target of 8 weeks) (**Fig. 1**).

Similarly to the Canadian study, the primar determinant of neck dissection was standar CT criteria of positive nodes. However, treatin

Table 1
Effectiveness of PET versus CT in decision making for neck dissection

Study	Moeller[40]	Porceddu[41]	Waldron[42]	Thariat[28]
Design	Prospective single-institution cohort	Prospective single-institution cohort	Prospective multi-institution cohort	Retrospective single-institution cohort
Population	All patients with stage III–IVB HNSCC[a,b]	All patients with N+ HNSCC with complete response at primary site	All patients with HNSCC and N2 or N3 disease	All patients with N+ HNSCC[b]
Treatment	Definitive radiotherapy ± chemotherapy	Definitive radiotherapy ± chemotherapy	Definitive radiotherapy ± chemotherapy	Definitive radiotherapy ± chemotherapy
Assessment of Response	^{18}FDG-PET at 8 wk	^{18}FDG-PET at 12 wk[c]	^{18}FDG-PET at 8–10 wk	CT at 4–8 wk
Number	98	112	399	880
T0 (%)	4	4	15	0
T1-T2 (%)	36	49	48	52
T3-T4 (%)	60	46	37	48
N0 (%)	18	0	0	0
N1 (%)	13.0	12.5	0.0	23.0
N2 (%)	66	75	90	71
N3 (%)	1.0	12.5	10.0	6.0
Primary site				
unknown (%)	0	4	0	0
Nasopharynx (%)	0	9	0	0
Oropharynx (%)	79	74	75	77
Oral cavity (%)	0	0	9	0
Hypopharynx (%)	12	6	8	9
Larynx (%)	9	6	8	14
HPV positive[d] (%)	Not stated	53	Not stated	Not stated
Neck dissections	20 (20%)	8 (7%)	152 (38%)	268 (30%)
Positive neck dissections	4/20 (20%)	6/8 (75%)	51/152 (34%)	80/268 (30%)
Length of follow-up	80% >18 mo	Median 28 mo	Median 92 wk	Median 51 mo
Overall survival	89%	88%	Not stated	Not stated
Number of nodal failures	4 (4.0%)	5 (4.5%)	4/201[e] (4.0%)	105 (12.0%)
Isolated neck failures	0 (0%)	2 (2%)	Not stated	30 (4%)

This table summarizes the findings from the prospective studies on the use of PET to make decisions about neck dissection after chemoradiation for head and neck cancer and compares them with the largest study evaluating the use of PET.
Abbreviations: N1, node positive; N2, single node >3 cm or multiple nodes (unilateral or bilateral); N3, any node >6 cm.
[a] American Joint Cancer Classification, sixth edition.
[b] Limited to oropharynx, hypopharynx, and larynx.
[c] Repeated at 16 weeks for equivocal cases.
[d] By positive expression for p-16.
[e] Data only presented for those not undergoing neck dissection.

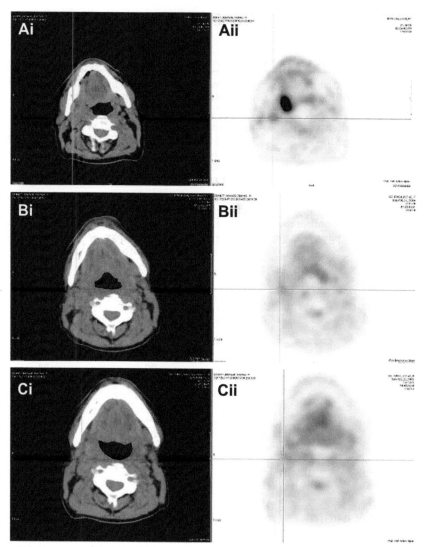

Fig. 1. Serial scans of 76-year-old man diagnosed with T3 N2c HPV-related oropharyngeal cancer. (*A*) pretreatment CT (*i*) and PET (*ii*) components of scan identifying primary tumor and ipsilateral level IIa lymph node. (*B*) CT (*i*) and PET (*ii*) components of scan 12 weeks after completion of treatment. Note complete response at primary site but low-grade FDG avidity at site of lymph node that was classed as equivocal. (*C*) CT (*i*) and PET (*ii*) components of scan 16 weeks after completion of treatment with resolution of changes at nodal site.

physicians had the discretion of using other criteria, such as increased PET avidity alone.

Patients were labeled as either *responders* or *nonresponders* to radiotherapy as determined by subsequent recurrence (either pathologically or clinically). Crucially, in their analysis of the utility of PET compared with CT, they did not distinguish between failure in the neck or other sites. They concluded that PET provided little value above CT in assigning response.

Brisbane Study

In the series by Porceddu and colleagues,[41] a cohort of patients was followed prospectively

after radiotherapy with or without chemotherapy for HNSCC using a defined PET-directed protocol. Only those with a complete response at the primary site based on a multidisciplinary assessment of clinical, radiological (CT and/or MR imaging), and PET-CT at 12 weeks were eligible.

The policy mandated that those with a complete PET response at the nodal site should be observed regardless of CT findings. Those with equivocal responses went on to have a repeat PET at 16 weeks. Patients with a positive PET at 12 weeks or an equivocal or positive PET at 16 weeks were referred for a neck dissection at the earliest possible date.

The median follow-up for the study was 28 months. An important finding was that only 2 isolated nodal failures occurred during the study, giving a 2-year isolated nodal failure rate of 2% (95% confidence interval, 1%–9%), which compares favorably with other studies using CT only[11,28,29] and supports the safety of this policy in clinical practice.

Of note is the fact that both failures occurred in the 8 patients who were PET positive and who underwent neck dissection. Of all the patients who were PET negative (103) and observed, none experienced an isolated neck failure (although 2 did fail at the primary or metastatic sites at the same time as a nodal failure). Also of note is that 6 out of the 8 (75%) neck dissections were positive for cancer cells.

In addition, this is the only study, as part of a defined PET-directed policy, to mandate a second scan when the initial is equivocal. As discussed later, the timing of PET is likely to have implications with its accuracy. It should be noted that 10 out of the 11 equivocal scans appropriately became negative on the repeat scan, suggesting that that earlier scanning can result in false positivity.

The most important finding from this study was the number of patients that were saved from neck dissection and the resultant morbidity. Only 8 (7%) patients underwent neck dissection. If a policy of planned neck dissection in N2 or N3 disease was used, then 98 (87.5%) patients would have undergone surgery with no difference in outcome. If a CT-guided policy was used, then 50 (45%) patients would have undergone surgery.

Canadian Study

The study by Waldron and colleagues[42] has only been presented in abstract form. It was a prospective multicenter study performed in patients with N2 or N3 HNSCC treated curatively with radiotherapy with or without chemotherapy. Contrast-enhanced CT scans and PET-CT were performed before and after treatment. At 8 to 10 weeks, the optimum timing of the posttreatment scan was earlier than the Brisbane study but similar to the MD Anderson study.

In contrast to the Brisbane study, the decision to undergo neck dissection was based solely on the presence of residual nodes greater than 1 cm in axial dimension on CT, and there was no scope to repeat imaging in equivocal cases.

Crucially, the assessment of the usefulness of PET was based on its correlation to histopathologic findings in those undergoing neck dissection rather than the clinical outcome of neck node failure.

A total of 399 patients were enrolled with similar subsite and T and N classifications as the other groups, although no N1 disease was allowed in this trial. A total of 353 patients underwent a PET-CT scan at a median of 9 weeks but as early as 4 weeks. One hundred fifty-one (43%) of these went on to have a neck dissection, with 50 out of 151 (33%) having positive histopathology. PET-CT had a sensitivity of 54%, specificity of 66%, PPV 44%, and NPV 74% when compared with the pathologic findings. Of the 202 patients who did not have neck dissection, 4% had neck recurrence on follow-up. They concluded that PET-CT was not a reliable indicator of residual nodal disease and should not be used to determine the need for neck dissection.

Comparison of Prospective PET Studies

Both the Canadian and MD Anderson studies conclude that the addition of PET did not add to the utility of standard CT evaluation, whereas the Brisbane study found that PET was extremely useful in reducing the number of patients with residual neck nodes.

There are some significant differences in how the studies were designed and in the results they produced, which are relevant to any discussion about the usefulness of PET. The following sections discuss these differences and may explain the contrasting conclusions about the usefulness of PET.

Population

A possible explanation could be different patient populations with differing risks of failure. However, this is unlikely given that these were all unselected populations undergoing standard therapy in modern centers. Indeed, the demographic data presented show similar patterns between the 3 studies: most patients are male; the median age is in the sixth decade; most tumors are of the oropharynx, of similar range of size, and of similar nodal states; and similar smoking history. Of note is the fact that the Brisbane study is the only study to try to identify the rate of HPV-associated disease, with 71% of oropharyngeal tumors HPV related. This figure alone represents 53% of the whole population.

Timing of PET/Protocol for Equivocal Results

In both the MD Anderson and Canadian studies, most patients underwent PET scanning around week 8 to 9, with some as early as 4 weeks. This practice was to facilitate neck dissection in a timely fashion when it was required. However, in the Brisbane study, after a clinical examination at 6 weeks to ensure nodes were not enlarging, the aim was for the PET scan to take place after 12 weeks, with a repeat at 16 weeks for equivocal cases. A repeat scan was performed in 11 patients; 10 patients were able to successfully avoid neck dissection because the repeat PET scan was negative.

There is evidence that the timing of the scan does affect the accuracy of the result with PET.[34–39,44,45] Greven and colleagues[45] demonstrated that PET at 4 months after the completion of therapy was more accurate than PET at 1 month. It is conceivable that the differing results can be partly explained by the early timing of the PET scan in the Canadian and MD Anderson studies compared with the later initial scan plus the option of a second scan in equivocal cases in the Brisbane study.

As always, the dilemma still exists between trying to avoid surgery in the majority that ultimately do not require it versus not wanting to delay surgery in those that do. Although the optimum approach is not yet certain, a later (12 weeks) rather than earlier (8 week) PET scan may be a pragmatic compromise. The policy of an additional scan at 16 weeks for the few cases that are equivocal may further increase the accuracy of PET by successfully avoiding surgery in most cases without a significant delay in the few when it is required.

Definition of PET Positivity

Although PET is a potentially quantitative measure of metabolic and, hence, malignant activity, there is not always direct correlation between measures of tracer uptake (typically maximum standardized uptake [SUV_{max}]) and malignancy. Although cutoff values of SUV_{max} of 2.5 to 3.0 have been reported as having high sensitivity and specificity for residual malignancy after chemoradiation,[34,35] others[37] have not found specific SUV cutoffs helpful. Issues, such as variations in physiologic uptake; asymmetry; or reduced volume, such as a residual rim of malignant cells in a necrotic tumor, can cause difficulty in interpreting scans before treatment. These difficulties are potentially even greater after treatment. Fuki and colleagues[46] showed how correlating the structural anatomic data from the CT component with the metabolic information from the PET component of a dedicated PET-CT scanner can help account for these issues and potentially reduce the pitfalls of relying solely on SUV. All 3 studies used conventional dedicated PET-CT scans. However, it is clear that a high degree of expertise is required in reporting scans.

In the study from Brisbane, scans were reported independently by 2 qualified nuclear medicine physicians with positivity related to focal uptake in structural abnormalities referenced to background activity in the liver rather than specific SUV. In equivocal cases, the scan was repeated at 16 weeks. All but one repeat scan was negative. In the study from MD Anderson, a single experienced nuclear medicine physician reported scans and referenced results with a value of SUV_{max}. PET reporting from the Canadian study was on a 5-point scale, with borderline cases considered positive.

It is possible that differences in reporting results, particularly about equivocal/borderline cases, may partially explain the differences between studies. The limitation of studies performed in only a few centers by a handful of reporters means that the whole-scale application of these policies should be done cautiously. However, this is also true of the accepted data on CT,[27–29] which come from single-institution studies. The results of the multi-institutional UK based PET-NECK study may help address this issue.

End Point

It is not surprising that the differing end points chosen in the 3 studies has led to differing interpretation as to the usefulness of PET. The Brisbane study used the clinical end point of isolated nodal relapse in a group of patients who had shown a complete response at the primary site to radiotherapy. It is this group alone that may potentially benefit from a planned neck dissection. Conversely, those who do not fail or who fail at other sites (primary or metastatic) either alone or at the same time as in the neck are unlikely to benefit from planned neck dissection but are at risk of its complications.

Because no isolated nodal failures occurred in the group that avoided neck dissection, the value of PET was in reducing the number of neck dissection from 50 that would have occurred with a CT directed policy to 8 with a PET-guided policy. Because the only 2 isolated nodal failures occurred in those who had already undergone neck dissection, even performing a planned neck dissection on all patients would not have reduced the failure rate.

The Canadian study and the MD Anderson study used pathologic and composite clinicopathologic end points, respectively. It is known that there is a poor correlation between the rate of positive pathologic specimens in series with planned neck dissections (up to 40%)[17,18] and the rate of subsequent nodal failure in complete responders from observation studies (less than 5%).[11,28,2] Therefore, the failure of PET to identify patients

ith positive histology does not mean that the PET
:an failed to identify a patient who would benefit
ɔm a planned neck dissection.

Also, the study by Moeller[40] was designed to
valuate the utility of PET in the assessment of
sponse to chemoradiation rather than the
ɔecific question of its role in managing the neck
ter treatment. Of its 98 patients, 16 were either
ɜnsored or labeled as nonresponders because
the development of metastatic disease or simul-
neous failure in the neck and other sites. None of
ese would have been saved by a planned neck
ssection. Although this article provides useful
formation on the utility of PET in assessing
sponse to chemoradiation, its conclusions
ɪould be used with caution when addressing
ɪe specific question of the usefulness of PET in
ɜtermining the value of a planned neck dissection
ter complete response at the primary site.

Perhaps the most telling fact when comparing
ɪe 3 studies is the very low isolated neck recur-
ɜnce rate (<5%) in all but the different rate of
ɜck dissection: 8% when decisions were based
n CT-PET at 12 weeks (with an option to repeat
t 16 weeks in equivocal cases) compared with
3% and 24% when decisions were based on
T at around 8 to 9 weeks.

isk Stratification?

could be argued that the high rates of oropharyn-
ɜal cancer, including HPV-related tumors (see
able 1), means that patients from these studies
re predominantly from low to intermediate risk
ɾoups whereby the rate of neck relapse would
ɜ expected to be low. However, these are unse-
ɜcted groups and reflect the patients coming
ɪrough modern head and neck clinics.[7] If a higher
ɾoportion of patients in modern practice come
ɔm good prognosis groups, it lends more weight
ɔ using a policy that can safely eliminate unneces-
ary neck dissection for the majority while allowing
to take place at the appropriate time for the few
ʌho may benefit.

What is uncertain is whether patients at greater
ɪsk of treatment failure (nonoropharynx, HPV-
ɜgative tumors) benefit equally because these
ɪake up only a small proportion of the cohorts.
he CT-directed study by Thariat[28] showed that
atients with tumors of the hypopharynx and
ɪrynx had worse outcomes, especially if they
Iso had enlarged lymph nodes. However, this
ɪay be because they had less chance of
complete response to therapy. What is unclear
ɜ whether patients with tumors at these subsites
re equally well served by a PET-directed policy
ɔward neck dissection. However, subset analysis

of the study by Moller[40] suggests that the accuracy of PET was increased in higher-risk groups
and that this was because of its ability to identify
residual nodal disease.

Midtherapy PET

In addition to assessing the response after the
completion of treatment, there is some evidence
that performing a PET during treatment may be
useful in predicting response. In a series of 47
patients evaluated by Brun and colleagues,[47]
lower avidity on an FDG-PET 1 to 3 weeks into
a course of radiotherapy correlated well with
both overall survival and local control. However,
in a study by Lee and colleagues,[48] the use of
the hypoxia marker [^{18}F]–misonidazole as a PET
tracer did not show correlation between midtreatment scans and patient outcomes. Although it is
tempting to speculate that a midtreatment scan
would be useful in identifying those at high risk of
residual nodal disease so that a planned neck
dissection could be performed soon after completion of treatment, there is little evidence to back up
this policy, especially because this may subject
those with the poorest outcome (incomplete
response at the primary site) to a futile neck
dissection.

Cost-Effectiveness

There have been several recent attempts to identify the optimum strategy by modeling the costs
of various strategies for managing the neck after
chemoradiation. Sher and colleagues[49] have
recently published a cost-effectiveness analysis
comparing 3 strategies in the management of
a 50-year-old man with a locally advance HNSCC.

- Planned neck dissection
- A CT stratified approach
- A PET-CT stratified approach

Although a theoretical exercise, it used a wide
range of realistic and exaggerated circumstance
to assess both the direct and indirect costs,
including those related to toxicity or salvage therapies, over the 5 years following the initial treatment. The PET-CT strategy consistently came
out as the most cost-effective and was also associated with more quality-adjusted life-years largely
because of the reduction in the amount of neck
dissection performed.

Rabalais and colleagues[50] compared the costs
of a planned neck dissection with a strategy of
serial PET-CT scans over the first year of treatment
in a patient with N2 neck disease. This study was
limited to the financial costs incurred in a US

setting and again indicated that a PET-CT policy (using up to 4 scans) was more cost-effective.

Cost-effectiveness analysis of the data published from the Brisbane series[41] (David Pryor, MBBS, Brisbane, QLD, Australia, personal communication, April 2012) again suggests that, when direct financial costs alone are considered, in an Australian setting, a PET-CT policy is more cost-effective than either planned neck dissection or CT-directed policies.

Although the 3 studies have used different assumptions and strategies in their modeling, the consistent finding of cost savings and improvements in quality of life support the use of PET-CT in decision making around the management of the neck following chemoradiation.

One criticism of the published cost-effectiveness data is direct comparison of planned neck dissection with either a CT or a PET-CT policy alone. Because it is known that a complete response at 6 to 8 weeks on clinical examination and CT is highly predictive of a low risk of isolated nodal relapse,[11,28,29] it could be argued that the additional cost of a PET-CT for these patients is unnecessary. Therefore, a combined strategy of routine CT scan and clinical evaluation at 6 weeks followed by PET-CT at 12 weeks only for those with a positive CT may, in fact, turn to be the most cost-effective. Indeed, the analysis of Brisbane data by Prior described earlier suggests that such a policy may be slightly more cost-effective. **Fig. 2** illustrates such a hypothetical policy. More patient

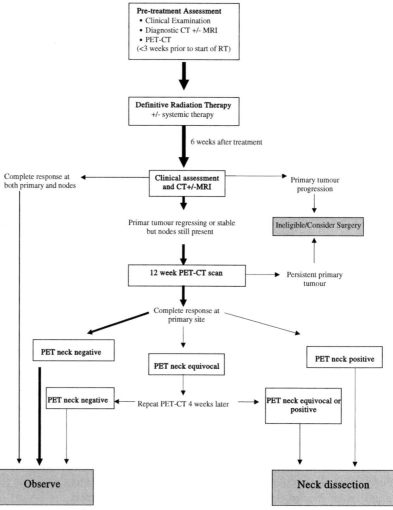

Fig. 2. Hypothetical optimum strategy managing the neck after chemoradiation. *Arrows leaving each text box represents possible outcomes at that point. So at the 6 week clinical/CT/MRI assessment there are 3 possible outcomes - complete response - progressive disease - and partial response. Each of the arrows leaving this box follow the pathway that each response results in. Thicker arrow represents more patients likely to follow that particular pathway. RT, radiation therapy.

likely to follow pathways with thicker arrows. However, it must be pointed out that this approach has not been prospectively validated. In addition, the proportion of patients who are complete responders by CT and clinical assessment and, hence, spared PET-CT may be as low as 25%.[27] The additional clinical workload of CT and PET-CT for the majority in this 2-stage approach may be clinically less appealing than a simple 1-stage PET-CT approach.

SUMMARY

- The management of the neck after chemo-radiation for HNSCC continues to evolve because of improvements in treatment modalities, the changing biology of the disease, and improvements in our ability to assess the response.
- As control rates improve and patients survive for longer periods after treatment, it is important that we limit the burden of long-term toxicity on both patients and society as a whole.
- Currently, PET-CT performed 12 weeks after completion of chemoradiation seems to be a useful tool in this decision-making process. Those patients who have achieved a complete response at the primary site but who retain structural nodal abnormalities on CT may be safely spared a potentially debilitating neck dissection if the PET-CT shows no metabolic abnormality.
- Despite the initial cost, a strategy of routine PET-CT may, in fact, be the most clinically useful and cost-effective strategy because of both the direct surgical savings and the reduction in the long-term costs of toxicity.

REFERENCES

1. National Comprehensive Cancer Network (NCCN) clinical practice guideline in oncology. Head and neck cancers. Version 2.2011. Available at: http://www.nccn.org/professionals/physician_gls/pdf/head-and neck.pdf. Accessed April 4, 2012.
2. Hamoi M, Ferlito A, Schmitz S, et al. The role of neck dissection in the setting of chemoradiation therapy for head and neck squamous cell carcinoma with advanced neck disease. Oral Oncol 2012;48:203–10.
3. Pignon P, Le Maître A, Maillard E, et al. Meta-analysis of chemotherapy in head and neck cancer (MACH-NC): an update on 93 randomised trials and 17,346 patients. Radiother Oncol 2009;92:4–14.
4. Fu KK, Pajak TF, Trotti A, et al. A Radiation Therapy Oncology Group (RTOG) phase III randomized study to compare hyperfractionation and two variants of accelerated fractionation to standard fractionation radiotherapy for head and neck squamous cell carcinomas: first report of RTOG 9003. Int J Radiat Oncol Biol Phys 2000;48:7–16.
5. Overgaard J, Hansen HS, Specht L, et al. Five compared with six fractions per week of conventional radiotherapy of squamous-cell carcinoma of head and neck: DAHANCA 6 and 7 randomised controlled trial. Lancet 2003;362:933–40.
6. Skladowski K, Maciejewski B, Golen M, et al. Continuous accelerated 7-days-a-week radiotherapy for head-and-neck cancer: long-term results of phase III clinical trial. Int J Radiat Oncol Biol Phys 2006;66:706–13.
7. Sturgis EM, Ang KK. The epidemic of HPV-associated oropharyngeal cancer is here: is it time to change our treatment paradigms? J Natl Compr Canc Netw 2011;9:665–73.
8. Lavertu P, Bonafede JP, Adelstein DJ, et al. Comparison of surgical complications after organ-preservation therapy in patients with stage III or IV squamous cell head and neck cancer. Arch Otolaryngol Head Neck Surg 1998;124:401–6.
9. Machtay M, Moughan J, Trotti A, et al. Factors associated with severe late toxicity after concurrent chemoradiation for locally advanced head and neck cancer: an RTOG analysis. J Clin Oncol 2008;26:3582–9.
10. Donatelli-Lassig AA, Duffy SA, Fowler KE, et al. The effect of neck dissection on quality of life after chemoradiation. Otolaryngol Head Neck Surg 2008;139:511–8.
11. Corry J, Peters L, Fisher R, et al. N2-N3 neck nodal control without planned neck dissection for clinical/radiological complete responders – results of Trans Tasman Radiation Oncology Group Study 98.02. Head Neck 2008;30:737–42.
12. Barkley HT Jr, Fletcher GH, Jesse RH, et al. Management of cervical lymph node metastases in squamous cell carcinoma of the tonsillar fossa, base of tongue, supraglottic larynx, and hypopharynx. Am J Surg 1972;124:462–7.
13. Carinci F, Cassano L, Farina A, et al. Unresectable primary tumor of head and neck: does neck dissection combined with chemoradiotherapy improve survival? J Carinofac Surg 2001;12:438–43.
14. Mendenhall WM, Parsons JT, Mancuso AA, et al. Head and neck: management of the neck. In: Perez CA, Brady LW, editors. Principles and practice of radiation oncology. 2nd edition. Philadelphia: J.B. Lippincott; 1992. p. 790–805.
15. Ellis ER, Mendenhall WM, Rao PV, et al. Incisional or excisional neck-node biopsy before definitive radiotherapy, alone or followed by neck dissection. Head Neck 1991;13:177–83.
16. Frank DK, Hu KS, Culliney BE, et al. Planned neck dissection after concomitant radiochemotherapy

for advance head and neck cancer. Laryngoscope 2005;115:1015–20.

17. Lavertu P, Adelstein DJ, Saxon JP, et al. Management of the neck in a randomised trial comparing concurrent chemotherapy and radiotherapy with radiotherapy alone in resectable stage III and IV squamous cell head and neck cancer. Head Neck 1997;19:559–66.

18. Stenson KM, Haraf DJ, Pelzer H, et al. The role of cervical lymphadenectomy after aggressive concomitant chemoradiotherapy: the feasibility of selective neck dissection. Arch Otolaryngol Head Neck Surg 2000;126:950–6.

19. Wolf GT, Fisher SG. Effectiveness of salvage neck dissection for advanced regional metastases when induction chemotherapy and radiation are used for organ preservation. Laryngoscope 1992;102:934–e939.

20. Mabanta SR, Mendenhall WM, Stringer SP, et al. Salvage treatment for neck recurrence after irradiation alone for head and neck squamous cell carcinoma with clinically positive neck nodes. Head Neck 1999;21:591–4.

21. Bernier J, Bataini JP. Regional outcome in oropharyngeal and pharyngolaryngeal cancer treated with high dose per fraction radiotherapy. Analysis of neck disease response in 1646 cases. Radiother Oncol 1986;6:87–103.

22. Mendenhall WM, Million RR, Cassisi NJ. Squamous cell carcinoma of the head and neck treated with radiation therapy: the role of neck dissection for clinically positive neck nodes. Int J Radiat Oncol Biol Phys 1986;12:733–40.

23. Mendenhall WM, Villaret DB, Amdur RJ, et al. Planned neck dissection after definitive radiotherapy for squamous cell carcinoma of the head and neck. Head Neck 2002;24:1012–8.

24. Paximadis PA, Christensen ME, Dyson G, et al. Upfront neck dissection followed by concurrent chemoradiation in patients with regionally advanced head and neck cancer. Head Neck 2012. http://dx.doi.org/10.1002/hed.22011. [Epub ahead of print].

25. Prades JM, Timoshenko AP, Schmitt TH, et al. Planned neck dissection before combined chemoradiation for pyriform sinus carcinoma. Acta Otolaryngol 2008;128:324–8.

26. Wong LY, Wei WI, Lam LK, et al. Salvage of recurrent head and neck squamous cell carcinoma after primary curative surgery. Head Neck 2003;25:953–9.

27. Ojiri H, Mendenhall WM, Stringer SP, et al. Post-RT CT results as a predictive model for the necessity of planned post-RT neck dissection in patients with cervical metastatic disease from squamous cell carcinoma. Int J Radiat Oncol Biol Phys 2002;52:420–8.

28. Thariat J, Ang KK, Allen PK, et al. Prediction of neck dissection requirement after definitive radiotherapy for head and neck squamous cell carcinoma. J Radiat Oncol Biol Phys 2012;82:e367–74.

29. Peters LJ, Weber RS, Morrison, et al. Neck surgery patients with primary oropharyngeal cancer treated with radiotherapy. Head Neck 1996;18:552–9.

30. Van der Putten I, Van der Broek GB, De Bree R, et Effectiveness of salvage selective and modified radical neck dissection for regional pathologic lymphadenopathy after chemoradiation. Head Neck 2009;31:593–603.

31. De Bondt RB, Nelemans PJ, Hofman PA, et al. Detection of lymph node metastases in head and neck cancer: a meta-analysis comparing US, USgFNA, CT and MR imaging. Eur J Radiol 2007;64:266–72.

32. Blodgett TM, Fukui MB, Snyderman CH, et al. Combined PET-CT in the head and neck part Physiologic, altered physiologic, and artifactual FDG uptake. Radiographics 2005;25:897–912.

33. Branstetter BF, Blodgett TM, Zimmer LA, et al. PET/CT more accurate than Pet or CT alone? Radiology 2005;235:580–6.

34. Yao M, Graham MM, Hoffman HT, et al. The role of post radiation therapy FDG-PET in prediction of necessity for post-radiation therapy neck dissection in locally advanced head-and-neck squamous cell carcinoma Int J Radiat Oncol Biol Phys 2004;59:1001–10.

35. Yao M, Smith RB, Graham MM, et al. The role of FDG PET in management of neck metastasis from head and-neck cancer after definitive radiation treatment Int J Radiat Oncol Biol Phys 2005;63:991–9.

36. Porceddu SV, Jarmolowski E, Hicks RJ, et al. Utility of positron emission tomography for the detection of disease in residual neck nodes after (chemo) radiotherapy in head and neck cancer. Head Neck 2005;27:175–81.

37. Ong SC, Schöder H, Lee NY, et al. Clinical utility of 18F-FDG PET/CT in assessing the neck after concurrent chemoradiotherapy for locoregional advanced head and neck cancer. J Nucl Med 2008;49:532–40.

38. Zundel MT, Michel MA, Schultz CJ, et al. Comparison of physical examination and fluorodeoxyglucose positron emission tomography/computed tomography 4-6 months after radiotherapy to assess residual head and neck cancer. Int J Radiat Oncol Biol Phys 2011;81:e825–32.

39. Nayak JV, Walvekar RR, Andrade RS, et al. Deferring planned neck dissection following chemoradiation for stage IV head and neck cancer: the utility of PET-CT. Laryngoscope 2007;117:2129–34.

40. Moeller BJ, Rana V, Cannon BA, et al. Prospective risk-adjusted [18F] fluorodeoxyglucose positron emission tomography and computed tomography assessment of radiation response in head & neck cancer. J Clin Oncol 2009;27:2509–15.

41. Porceddu SV, Pryor DI, Burmeister E. Results of a prospective study of positron emission tomography directed management of residual nodal abnormalities

in node-positive head and neck cancer after definitive radiotherapy with or without systemic therapy. Head Neck 2011;33:1675–82.

. Waldron JN, Gilbert RW, Eapen L, et al. Results of an Ontario Clinical Oncology Group (OCOG) prospective cohort study on the use of FDG PET/ CT to predict the need for neck dissection following radiation therapy of head and neck cancer (HNC). ASCO Meeting Abstracts 2011; 29(Suppl 15):5504.

3. PET-NECK study Summary. UK Clinical Research Network: portfolio database. Available at: http://public. ukcrn.org.uk/search/StudyDetail.aspx?StudyID=3799. Accessed April 4, 2012.

. Gourin CG, Williams HT, Seabolt WN, et al. Utility of positron emission tomography-computed tomography in identification of residual nodal disease after chemoradiation for advanced head and neck cancer. Laryngoscope 2006;116:705–10.

5. Greven KM, Williams DW 3rd, McGuirt WF Sr, et al. Serial positron emission tomography scans following radiation therapy of patients with head and neck cancer. Head Neck 2001;23:942–6.

46. Fukui MB, Blodgett TM, Snyderman CH, et al. Combined PET-CT in the head and neck part 2. diagnostic uses and pitfalls of oncologic imaging. Radiographics 2005;25:913–30.

47. Brun E, Kjellén E, Tennvall J, et al. FDG PET studies during treatment: prediction of therapy outcomes in head and neck squamous cell carcinoma. Head Neck 2002;24:127–35.

48. Lee N, Nehmeh S, Schöder H, et al. Prospective trial incorporating pre-/mid-treatment [18f]-misonidazole positron emission tomography for head-and-neck cancer patients undergoing concurrent chemoradio-therapy. Int J Radiat Oncol Biol Phys 2009;75:101–8.

49. Sher DJ, Tishler RB, Annino D, et al. Cost-effective-ness of CT and PET-CT for determining the need for adjuvant neck dissection in locally advanced head and neck cancer. Ann Oncol 2010;21:1072–7.

50. Rabalais A, Walvekar RR, Johnson JT, et al. A cost-effectiveness analysis of positron emission tomography-computed tomography surveillance versus up-front neck dissection for management of the neck for N2 disease after chemoradiotherapy. Laryngoscope 2012;122(2):311–4.

Newer Methods for Improving Yield from FDG-PET Imaging for Accurate Staging, Determining Tumor Biology, and Assessing Prognosis

Roland Hustinx, MD, PhD

KEYWORDS

• Head and neck • FDG • PET/CT • Dual time point • Acquisition protocol

KEY POINTS

- Dual time point FDG PET imaging may improve the diagnostic accuracy and prognostic characterization of head and neck squamous cell carcinoma.
- Dedicated acquisition and reconstruction algorithms clearly enhance the diagnostic performance of FDG PET/CT.
- In squamous cell carcinoma, a survey limited to the head and neck area, chest, and upper abdomen is clinically acceptable. Nasopharyngeal carcinoma requires a whole-body study.

Fluorodeoxyglucose (FDG) PET/CT is a powerful tool for staging head and neck cancer at diagnosis and after treatment, and for evaluating the response to treatment. It also provides valuable prognostic information. The term "head and neck cancer" comprises carcinomas arising in the lip; oral cavity; oropharynx; hypopharynx; nasopharynx; glottic and supraglottic larynx; paranasal ethmoid and maxillary) sinuses; and salivary glands. More than 95% of head and neck cancers are squamous cell carcinoma (HNSCC); tobacco abuse and alcohol are common etiologic factors. Human papillomavirus is a newer causal factor for subtypes of HNSCC.[1] Forty percent of HNSCC are at early stage at the time of diagnosis (T1-2 N0) and the relative 5-year survival rate in the United States is 83%.[2] Sixty percent of patients present with advanced stage (stage III or IV) disease; most of these patients show locally advanced disease and metastases at diagnosis are uncommon. For patients with regional involvement and distant metastases, the 5-year survival rates drop to 54% and 32%, respectively.[2] Most distant

metastases and second primary cancers are found in the chest. One notable exception is the nasopharyngeal carcinoma, which has an entirely distinct natural history and shows a high propensity to disseminate to the skeleton.[3] Schematically, HNSCC may be considered as a tumor that, like all squamous cell carcinomas, displays consistently high avidity in FDG, with a high probability of locoregional spread and a relatively low probability of distant spread. Therefore, specific PET/CT acquisition protocols have been developed and tested to improve the performance of the technique in staging the disease and evaluating its prognosis.

DUAL TIME POINT IMAGING

It was recognized early on that FDG uptake in malignant tumors may not reach a plateau until several hours after injecting the tracer.[4,5] In 1999, Lodge and colleagues[6] showed that uptake in malignant soft tissue tumors did not plateau until 4 hours postinjection, whereas benign masses

Division of Nuclear Medicine, University Hospital of Liège, University of Liège, Sart Tilman, B35, Liège B-4000, Belgium
E-mail address: rhustinx@chu.ulg.ac.be

PET Clin 7 (2012) 425–430
http://dx.doi.org/10.1016/j.cpet.2012.06.005

and low-grade lesions reached their peak before 60 minutes. Animal experiments, however, had shown that the FDG uptake in turpentine oil–induced lesions reached its maximum after 60 minutes.[7] Based on these observations, the hypothesis was formed that a repeated FDG PET acquisition some minutes after the conventional whole-body study might help characterizing ambiguous foci of activity, by studying the evolution of the Standardized Uptake Value (SUV) over time. Initial results were highly encouraging. Twenty-one patients were serially scanned, with an average interval of 28 minutes between the two PET acquisitions.[8] Eighteen patients had a history of HNSCC and three were explored for osteomyelitis. Overall, a total of 18 cancerous lesions and nine inflammatory lesions were studied, along with normal structures in the head and neck area. Tumor SUVs increased by 12% compared with a 5% decrease for contralateral sites. SUVs for inflammatory sites, cerebellum, tongue, and larynx remained constant over time. The ratio tumor/contralateral SUV increased by 23% over time, whereas this ratio for inflamed sites increased by only 5%. The time interval between scans correlated with increase in SUV for tumors ($r = 0.55$; $P<.05$) but not for any of the other areas (**Fig. 1**). Separation was superior when studies were performed more than 30 minutes apart. Although encouraging, these data were obtained in a limited series of patients. Also, even though the results were statistically significant, the large standard deviations prevent using the changes in SUV for classifying the lesions on an individual basis. Wong and colleagues[9] further investigated the time sensitivity of head and neck tumors by performing dual time point FDG PET studies in 40 patients. The early and delayed scans were highly variable in time, with differences of 30 minutes on average in a group of patients and of 100 minutes in a second group. Through simple modeling, they found what they called the time

sensitivity factor (S) to be of value for reliably distinguishing the uptake kinetics in tumor and cerebellum. To date, no clinical application of this method has been reported. Conversely, in a series of 84 patients with nasopharyngeal carcinoma, delayed (3 hours) FDG scan did not improve the diagnostic performance of PET studies performed 4 minutes postinjection.[10] Considering the exceptionally high sensitivity (97.7%), specificity (94.9%), and accuracy (96.7%) of the early study, it is no wonder that decreasing the number of false-negative results from six to three, and the number of false-positive results from eight to seven, with the delayed scans did not significantly change the clinical results.

The prognostic value of dual time point FDG PET was studied in 12 patients with advanced HNSCC. The increase in SUV over time in the tumors was confirmed yet again and a trend toward predictive significance was noticed, although the sample was too limited to reach any definite conclusions.

DEDICATED ACQUISITION PROTOCOLS

The amount of radioactivity in structures whose size is less than twice the reconstructed image resolution is underevaluated by PET.[12] Using conventional whole-body protocols, modern PET scanners yield reconstructed images with a resolution of 5 to 8 mm. This takes into account the intrinsic spatial resolution of the system and the necessary smoothing to reduce image noise. Hence, the detection rate of lesions smaller than 10 mm is lower than that of larger lesions. It has been reported that more than 40% of the cervical nodal metastases occur in nodes that are no larger than 10 mm.[13] It makes perfect sense to try adapting the PET acquisition protocol to improve the detection rate of small lesions. This can be achieved by decreasing the pixel size in the reconstructed PET images. To maintain sufficient counting statistics and keep the noise at an acceptable

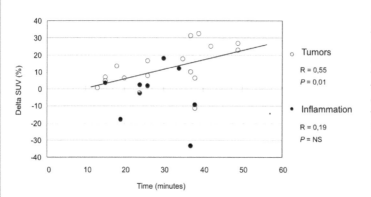

Fig. 1. Relationship between uptake time and changes in SUVs. (*Adapted from* Hustinx R, Smith RJ, Benard F, et al. Dual time point fluorine-18 fluorodeoxyglucose positron emission tomography: a potential method to differentiate malignancy from inflammation and normal tissue in the head and neck. Eur J Nucl Med 1999;26:1345; with permission.)

vel, the acquisition time has to be increased and e reconstruction parameters (filters, number of erations and subsets, and so forth) optimized.

cquisition Time and Pixel Size

amamoto and colleagues[14] performed studies sing a phantom about the same size as the neck an adult patient. A longer acquisition time minutes vs 2–4) yielded higher signal-to-noise tios, up to 27%. In patient studies, the dedicated ET acquisition time was 8 minutes, and the field view and pixel size of the reconstructed images ere 30 cm and 2.34 mm, respectively. Using the nventional protocol, the acquisition time was 2 4 minutes, depending on the body habitus of the atient; the field of view was 50 cm; and the pixel ze was 3.91 mm. In both cases, the matrix was 28 × 128. A total of 55 patients were included, ith a wide variety of tumor types. The reference andard was biopsy or clinical radiologic follow- . The SUVs in the primaries and in the lymph nodes ere significantly higher with the dedicated pro- col, which also revealed 11 nodes smaller than 1 m and not seen on the conventional PET images. egarding the diagnostic accuracy, however, there as no significant difference: the area under the eceiver operating characteristic curve (ROC) curve as 0.92 and 0.94 for the conventional and dedi- ated protocols, respectively.

ully Dedicated Protocols

odrigues and colleagues[15] further optimized dedicated protocol: the interval from FDG injec- on was increased to 150 minutes; the patient was laced on a flat bed with head in a holder; the cquisition time was doubled to 12 minutes per ed position; and the matrix was changed to 256 256, with a 1.5 zoom, so that the pixel size as 1.82 mm. The CT parameters were also nproved. They reviewed the data in 44 patients ith HNSCC who were considered candidates r curative surgery. The gold standard was histo- athology obtained by surgery, including unilateral r bilateral neck dissection. There was no signifi- ant difference for identifying the primary tumor: e dedicated protocol was slightly more sensitive 95% vs 92%) but less specific (83% vs 100%) han the whole-body protocol. Both were superior the contrast-enhanced CT (ceCT). Regarding /mph node metastases, the sensitivity, speci- city, accuracy, and positive predictive value and egative predictive value for the detection of nodal netastasis were 70%, 82%, 79%, 57%, and 89%, espectively, for the whole-body PET/CT protocol; 1%, 71%, 76%, 51%, and 96%, respectively, for he head and neck PET/CT protocol; and 57%,

88%, 81%, 63%, and 86%, respectively, for the ceCT protocol. ROC analysis showed that the head and neck protocol was significantly better than the whole-body protocol and ceCT on a per-level basis, but not on a per-patient basis. The primary advantage of the head and neck PET/CT protocol was the improved identification of involved lymph nodes smaller than 15 mm. As expected, the metabolic activity in the lymph no- des, as measured by the SUVs, was higher on the head and neck images compared with the whole-body images. A more than 10% increase in SUV was observed in 72% of the positive nodes and in 84% of the negative nodes. Following the whole-body PET/CT protocol, the mean SUVmax for positive nodes was 9.1 (range, 1.3–24), and the mean SUVmax for negative nodes was 2.8 (range, 0.6–6.5). Following the head and neck PET/CT protocol, the mean SUVmax for positive nodes was 10.4 (range, 1.1–31), and the mean SUVmax for negative nodes was 3 (range, 0.4– 9.6). With the whole-body protocol, 51% (18 of 35) of the positive nodes had metabolic activity that fell within the range of negative nodes, but this proportion increased to 66% (26 of 44) with the head and neck protocol. As a result, the very high negative predictive value (96%) comes at the cost of a slight decrease in specificity (71%) for the dedicated head and neck protocol. An example of improved resolution with a dedicated protocol is shown in **Fig. 2**.

Other refinements have been proposed, such as positioning the patient's head in a holder and using a bite device to keep the mouth open during the PET acquisition, which helps improve the precise anatomic location of oral cavity tumors.[16]

Contrast Enhancement

Considering the anatomic complexity of the head and neck area and the wide variety of normal structures that display variable FDG uptake in the absence of neoplastic involvement, one may expect better diagnostic results when using an optimized CT component of the PET/CT study. It is not clear whether ceCT really improves the over- all performances of FDG PET/CT in staging HNSCC. Yoshida and colleagues[17] prospectively studied 42 consecutive patients with previously untreated, biopsy-proved primary head and neck cancers. Contrast-enhanced and unenhanced PET/CT performed no differently, detecting 98% and 95% of the primary tumors, respectively, and 92% of patients with nodal disease for both techniques. Accuracy for T status was 75% and 73%, respectively, and 90% in both cases for the N status. According to these results, routine

A   B

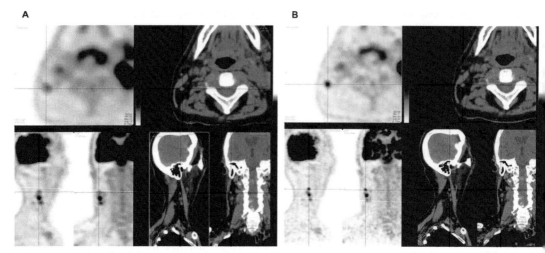

Fig. 2. Multiple lymph node metastases. The acquisition protocol was 4 minutes per bed position for the nec area and 1 minute for the reminder of the study. (*A*) Conventional whole-body reconstruction. The SUV in th upper lymph node (6 mm in largest diameter) was 3.1. (*B*) Dedicated high-resolution reconstruction protoco The images are a bit noisier but the contrast is higher, with an SUV of 6.8.

contrast enhancement of the CT part of the PET/CT does not seem useful. However, Haerle and colleagues[18] looked at the detection rate for necrotic lymph node metastases. They studied 34 patients with tonsillar SCC, whose lymph node metastases often take the form of cystic lesions, with a large proportion of necrosis.[19] This was a retrospective study, including patients with untreated tumors and selected for surgery as the first-line treatment. Pathologic analysis of the neck dissections was the gold standard. There was no statistical difference in terms of sensitivity, specificity, positive predictive value, negative predictive value, and accuracy of ceCT, PET/CT, and PET/ceCT with regard to correct pathologic nodal (pN) classification. The only difference was found when comparing PET/ceCT with PET alone. However, when the endpoint was distinguishing pN0 from pN+, the ROC-analysis showed a statistically significant difference between PET/ceCT and PET/CT, between PET/ceCT and PET alone, between ceCT and PET/CT, and between ceCT and PET alone, respectively. There was a negative linear correlation between the lymph node SUV and the grade of necrosis at pathologic analysis. In any case, even though contrast enhancement has not been proved mandatory in all cases, head and neck surgeons usually not only require a full-dose, contrast-enhanced, diagnostic CT but also an interpretation by an experienced radiologist, with the necessary expertise in this delicate field. The sole issue thus becomes whether such diagnostic CT is performed as part of the PET/CT study or separately.

Truncated Versus Whole-Body Acquisitions

Dedicated PET/CT acquisition protocols tha improve the diagnostic accuracy for nodal stagin imply increasing the scanning time over the nec area. Reducing the scan length by not scannin below the adrenals may present several advan tages, such as making up, at least partly, for th increased time spent over the neck, thus main taining the patient's throughput. Iagaru an colleagues[20] showed that the diagnostic yield o whole-body imaging is low in HNSCC, with onl 3% of significant findings below the level of th adrenal glands. Such a shortened imagin protocol cannot be applied to nasopahryngea carcinomas, however, because the yield wa significantly higher in this population (7.7%). A Australian study recently confirmed these finding in the posttreatment monitoring of HNSCC.[21] retrospective review of 240 patients with HNSC showed no occurrence of isolated disease belo the diaphragm, because all patients who devel oped metastases had lung lesions, in some case accompanied by liver lesions.

Newer Methods for Characterizing Tumor Metabolism

The clinical results of FDG PET/CT in stagin HNSCC are excellent, usually obtained throug a simple visual interpretation by an experience observer.[22,23] The SUV has also been propose as a prognostic indicator.[24] However, there ar ways to extract additional information from th PET/CT images, in addition to the visual analysi

d assessment of uptake intensity. A major field
investigation is the textural analysis of the PET
ages. The spatial heterogeneity, with the de-
rmination of such parameters as coarseness,
ontrast, busyness, or complexity, has been re-
ognized as predictive of outcome in several tu-
or types.[25,26] The method was applied for
elineating the tumor volume and distinguishing
mor from normal tissue in HNSCC.[27,28] Initial
sults are highly encouraging, because the me-
od described as a coregistered multimodality
attern analysis segmentation system was able to
stinguish cancer from adjacent normal tissues
ith high physiologic uptake and to consistently
efine tumors with large variability in FDG uptake
a small series of 10 patients.[28] In another set of
xperiments, the sensitivity and specificity for clas-
fying normal and abnormal tissue was 89% and
9%, respectively.[27] The clinical impact remains
nknown, but this approach is very attractive and
ay prove valuable as a prognostic tool and for
elping radiation oncologists define the target
olumes in a reliable and reproducible fashion.

EFERENCES

1. Argiris A, Karamouzis MV, Raben D, et al. Head and neck cancer. Lancet 2008;371:1695.
2. Jemal A, Siegel R, Xu J, et al. Cancer statistics. CA Cancer J Clin 2010;60:277.
3. Chiesa F, De Paoli F. Distant metastases from naso-pharyngeal cancer. ORL J Otorhinolaryngol Relat Spec 2001;63:214.
4. Hamberg LM, Hunter GJ, Alpert NM, et al. The dose uptake ratio as an index of glucose metabolism: useful parameter or oversimplification? J Nucl Med 1994;35:1308.
5. Fischman AJ, Alpert NM. FDG-PET in oncology: there's more to it than looking at pictures. J Nucl Med 1993;34:6.
6. Lodge MA, Lucas JD, Marsden PK, et al. A PET study of 18FDG uptake in soft tissue masses. Eur J Nucl Med 1999;26:22.
7. Yamada S, Kubota K, Kubota R, et al. High accumula-tion of fluorine-18-fluorodeoxyglucose in turpentine-induced inflammatory tissue. J Nucl Med 1995; 36:1301.
8. Hustinx R, Smith RJ, Benard F, et al. Dual time point fluorine-18 fluorodeoxyglucose positron emission tomography: a potential method to differentiate malignancy from inflammation and normal tissue in the head and neck. Eur J Nucl Med 1999;26:1345.
9. Wong CY, Noujaim D, Fu HF, et al. Time sensitivity: a parameter reflecting tumor metabolic kinetics by variable dual-time F-18 FDG PET imaging. Mol Imaging Biol 2009;11:283.
10. Yen TC, Chang YC, Chan SC, et al. Are dual-phase 18F-FDG PET scans necessary in nasopharyngeal carcinoma to assess the primary tumour and loco-regional nodes? Eur J Nucl Med Mol Imaging 2005;32:541.
11. Sanghera B, Wong WL, Lodge MA, et al. Potential novel application of dual time point SUV measure-ments as a predictor of survival in head and neck cancer. Nucl Med Commun 2005;26:861.
12. Hoffman EJ, Huang SC, Phelps ME. Quantitation in positron emission computed tomography: 1. Effect of object size. J Comput Assist Tomogr 1979;3:299.
13. van den Brekel MW, Stel HV, Castelijns JA, et al. Cervical lymph node metastasis: assessment of radiologic criteria. Radiology 1990;177:379.
14. Yamamoto Y, Wong TZ, Turkington TG, et al. Head and neck cancer: dedicated FDG PET/CT protocol for detection–phantom and initial clinical studies. Radiology 2007;244:263.
15. Rodrigues RS, Bozza FA, Christian PE, et al. Compar-ison of whole-body PET/CT, dedicated high-resolution head and neck PET/CT, and contrast-enhanced CT in preoperative staging of clinically M0 squamous cell carcinoma of the head and neck. J Nucl Med 2009; 50:1205.
16. Cistaro A, Palandri S, Balsamo V, et al. Assessment of a new 18F-FDG PET/CT protocol in the staging of oral cavity carcinomas. J Nucl Med Technol 2011;39:7.
17. Yoshida K, Suzuki A, Nagashima T, et al. Staging primary head and neck cancers with (18)F-FDG PET/CT: is intravenous contrast administration really necessary? Eur J Nucl Med Mol Imaging 2009; 36:1417.
18. Haerle SK, Strobel K, Ahmad N, et al. Contrast-enhanced (1)(8)F-FDG-PET/CT for the assessment of necrotic lymph node metastases. Head Neck 2011;33:324.
19. Thompson LD, Becker RC, Przygodzki RM, et al. Mucinous cystic neoplasm (mucinous cystadeno-carcinoma of low-grade malignant potential) of the pancreas: a clinicopathologic study of 130 cases. Am J Surg Pathol 1999;23:1.
20. Iagaru A, Mittra ES, Gambhir SS. FDG-PET/CT in cancers of the head and neck: what is the definition of whole body scanning? Mol Imaging Biol 2011; 13:362.
21. Huang YT, Ravi Kumar AS. Potential for truncating the scan length of restaging FDG-PET/CT after che-moradiotherapy in head and neck squamous cell carcinoma. Nucl Med Commun 2012;33:503.
22. Gupta T, Master Z, Kannan S, et al. Diagnostic performance of post-treatment FDG PET or FDG PET/CT imaging in head and neck cancer: a system-atic review and meta-analysis. Eur J Nucl Med Mol Imaging 2011;38:2083.
23. Xu GZ, Guan DJ, He ZY. (18)FDG-PET/CT for detect-ing distant metastases and second primary cancers

in patients with head and neck cancer. A meta-analysis. Oral Oncol 2011;47:560.

24. Xie P, Li M, Zhao H, et al. 18F-FDG PET or PET-CT to evaluate prognosis for head and neck cancer: a meta-analysis. J Cancer Res Clin Oncol 2011;137:1085.

25. Eary JF, O'Sullivan F, O'Sullivan J, et al. Spatial heterogeneity in sarcoma 18F-FDG uptake as a predictor of patient outcome. J Nucl Med 2008;49:1973.

26. Tixier F, Le Rest CC, Hatt M, et al. Intratumor heterogeneity characterized by textural features on baseline 18F-FDG PET images predicts response to concomitant radiochemotherapy in esophageal cancer. J Nucl Med 2011;52:369.

27. Yu H, Caldwell C, Mah K, et al. Coregistered FDG PET/CT-based textural characterization of head and neck cancer for radiation treatment planning. IEEE Trans Med Imaging 2009;28:374.

28. Yu H, Caldwell C, Mah K, et al. Automated radiation targeting in head-and-neck cancer using region-based texture analysis of PET and CT images. Int J Radiat Oncol Biol Phys 2009;75:618.

New Tracers PET in Head and Neck Squamous Cell Carcinoma

Tony J.C. Wang, MD[a], Yusuf Menda, MD[b],
Simon K. Cheng, MD, PhD[a], Cheng-Chia Wu, BS[a],
Nancy Y. Lee, MD[c],*

KEYWORDS

• PET • Head and neck cancer • Hypoxia • Fluoromisonidazole • Fluorothymidine

KEY POINTS

- We summarize new PET tracers that allow the biologic profiling of head and neck squamous cell carcinomas, such as hypoxia and cell proliferation.
- We discuss the latest studies on potential PET tracers for amino acid metabolism and specific molecular targets.
- We conclude with potential roles of new PET tracers to customize treatment for head and neck cancers.

INTRODUCTION

PET with [18F]fluorodeoxyglucose (FDG) in head and neck cancers is commonly used to provide biologic profiling as well as the staging of disease, whether a tumor has locoregional extension or metastatic spread.[1–5] FDG PET imaging of head and neck cancers is reviewed elsewhere in the issue by Min Yao and colleagues. In this review, we focus on new tracers for PET that assess tumor hypoxia, including [18F]fluoromisonidazole (FMISO), copper-diacetyl-bis(N4-methylthiosemicarbazone) (Cu-ATSM), and [18F]fluoroazomycin arabinoside (FAZA), and evaluate cell proliferation, with [18F]fluorothymidine (FLT), in head and neck squamous cell carcinoma (HNSCC). We also discuss tracers for assessing specific amino acid (AA) metabolism as well as epidermal growth factor receptor (EGFR) biomarkers. All of these radiopharmaceuticals are investigational and are not approved by the Food and Drug Administration for clinical use.

HYPOXIA

Several studies have shown that hypoxia occurs commonly in HNSCC.[6–8] Hypoxic tumors have been associated with poor clinical outcomes and are resistant to chemoradiation treatments.[7,9] It has been reported that hypoxic tumors require several times higher radiation doses to achieve the same level of cell killing compared with normoxic conditions.[10] Strategies to overcome hypoxia for HNSCC such as accelerated fractionation have not been promising.[11] Additionally, hypoxic tumors have resistance to many types of chemotherapies, including 5-fluorouracil, bleomycin, taxanes, doxorubicin, and etoposide.[12–17] Because of its poor prognostic implications, there has been much interest in imaging of hypoxia.[18,19] Early methods to detect hypoxia included invasive techniques such as directly measuring tumor oxygenation through oxygen electrodes. Newer methods include the

Conflict of interest: None.
[a] Department of Radiation Oncology, College of Physicians and Surgeons, Columbia University, 622 West 168th Street, New York, NY 10032, USA; [b] Department of Radiology, University of Iowa, 200 Hawkins Drive, Iowa City, IA, USA; [c] Department of Radiation Oncology, Memorial Sloan-Kettering Cancer Center, 1275 York Avenue, New York, NY 10065, USA
* Corresponding author.
E-mail address: leen2@mskcc.org

PET Clin 7 (2012) 431–441
http://dx.doi.org/10.1016/j.cpet.2012.06.009
1556-8598/12/$ – see front matter © 2012 Published by Elsevier Inc.

radiolabeling of hypoxia-specific compounds, which can be imaged with PET. The most commonly used hypoxia imaging agents are FMISO, FAZA and Cu-ATSM. FMISO has been most extensively studied in HNSCC.[10,20,21]

FMISO

FMISO is a nitroimidazole tracer that has been extensively studied at the University of Washington.[22–27] Under hypoxic conditions, FMISO, which is reduced and bound to cell constitutents, can depict the level of hypoxia.[28] FMISO PET has been studied in a variety of tumors, including lung cancer, prostate cancer, and head and neck cancer.[20,25,29–38] Rasey and colleagues[39] showed that human tumor hypoxia is very common and highly variable between tumors of the same histology and also between regions within the same tumor.

FMISO uptake in head and neck cancers correlates with Po_2 measurements using oxygen electrodes to assess tumor hypoxia in patients with HNSCC.[29] Eschmann and colleagues[20] reported that high uptake of FMISO in HNSCC could predict poor treatment outcome after radiotherapy. Furthermore, early resolution of FMISO uptake after treatment with a hypoxia targeting agent (tirapazamine) was associated with excellent locoregional control in advanced HNSCC.[30] Rajendran and colleagues[25] confirmed that pretreatment FMISO uptake showed a strong trend as an independent prognostic factor in HNSCC. In addition to primary tumors, FMISO uptake was correlated with hypoxia in metastatic neck nodes for HNSCC.[31]

One of the potential roles for FMISO is to evaluate the need to intensify treatment if tumor hypoxia is detected. Lee and colleagues[33] reported the first use of FMISO PET/computed tomography (CT)-guided intensity-modulated radiation therapy (IMRT) in which areas of hypoxia received a boost. The investigators showed that areas of hypoxia detected by FMISO could be dose escalated without compromising normal tissue sparing (**Fig. 1**). A subsequent prospective study by Lee and colleagues[32] assessed pretreatment and mid-treatment FMISO scans for patients with HNSCC undergoing chemoradiation therapy. Of the 20 patients who completed the protocol, 18 (90%) presented with pretreatment hypoxia on FMISO (**Fig. 2**). Of the 18 patients, 16 had complete resolution of hypoxia on the mid-treatment scan (**Fig. 3**). The authors reported that only 1 patient had persistent disease in the neck and subsequently developed distant metastasis. Surprisingly, this patient did not have positive FMISO uptake mid-treatment. A prospective study from

the Trans-Tasmanian Radiation Oncology Group Study reported that patients with HNSCC with pretreatment hypoxia detected by FMISO PET had higher risk of locoregional failure if as part of the chemoradiation therapy regimen they did not receive tirapazamine, a cytotoxin only activated under hypoxic conditions.[35]

One of the disadvantages of FMISO is the inherent variability of hypoxic volumes. Nehmeh and colleagues[34] showed that intratumoral FMISO distribution could vary between 2 scans that are days apart before radiation treatment in patients with HNSCC (**Fig. 4**). The results of these studies suggest that there may be a benefit for repeated FMISO PET scans during the course of radiation therapy for optimal localization of hypoxia within the tumor. There has been much interest in identifying the best model to quantify tumor hypoxia with FMISO.[36–38,40,41] In addition to standardized uptake value, lesion-to–normal organ ratios have been measured using tissue-to-muscle ratio and tissue-to-blood ratio.[24,36,42] Thorwarth and colleagues[36,37] developed a kinetic model to quantify hypoxia using FMISO and subsequently showed that combined FDG and FMISO data could improve assessment of local tumor characteristics. Wang and colleagues[38,41] used a plasma input 2-tissue irreversible compartment model combined with image-based plasma input function for analysis of FMISO data. Optimal studies to assess tumor hypoxia using FMISO are ongoing and we eagerly await the results.

Cu-ATSM

An alternative to FMISO for hypoxia imaging is Cu-ATSM. Cu-ATSM PET shows a higher tumor-to–background contrast ratio compared with FMISO.[43] Cellular uptake of Cu-ATSM, a lipophilic molecule, is proposed to be based on simple diffusion. Once inside the cell, it reacts with thiol groups or redox-active proteins with NADH as a cofactor. The reduced form of Cu-ATSM is more charged, thus causing cellular accumulation.[44] Several copper (Cu) isotopes can be used for ATSM labeling, including Cu-60, Cu-61, Cu-62, and Cu-64. Cu-60 and Cu-64 are the most commonly used copper isotopes for PET. Cu-60 has a half life of 23.7 minutes and Cu-64 has a half-life of 12.7 hours. Several studies have looked into incorporating Cu-ATSM for HNSCC treatment.[43,45–47] Chao and colleagues[45] used hypoxia imaging with Cu-ATSM to selectively dose-escalate hypoxic tumor subvolume by IMRT. Kositwattanarerk and colleagues[46] showed negative correlation between intratumoral uptake of FDG and Cu-ATSM in 27 patients with HNSCC

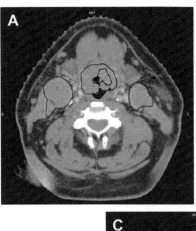
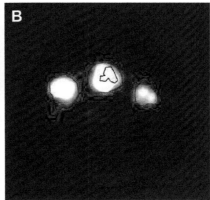
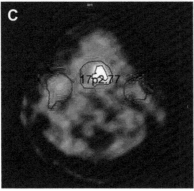

g. 1. Example of delineation of gross tumor volume and corresponding hypoxic gross tumor volume by FDG
ET/CT and FMISO PET/CT. (*A*) CT axial slice, (*B*) FDG-PET axial scan, and (*C*) FMISO PET axial slice. (*From* Lee NY,
Iechalakos JG, Nehmeh S, et al. Fluorine-18-labeled fluoromisonidazole positron emission and computed
omography-guided intensity-modulated radiotherapy for head and neck cancer: a feasibility study. Int J Radiat
Incol Biol Phys 2008;70:2–13; with permission.)

Iterestingly, there was a positive correlation with
Idenocarcinoma although the sample size was
mall. Minagawa and colleagues[47] reported in
pilot study of 15 patients that Cu-ATSM uptake
Iay predict tumor response to chemoradiation in
atients with HNSCC.

AZA

Inother compound used for hypoxia imaging, but
Iss studied for HNSCC, is FAZA. It is a nitroimida-
Iole compound like FMISO, but it seems to have
Ipid diffusion through tissue and faster renal
xcretion.[48] Grosu and Souvatzoglou reported
Ie first feasibility studies of FAZA as a hypoxia
Iarker in patients with HNSCC and its potential
se for IMRT dose-escalation.[49,50] A recent study
y Le and colleagues found a good correlation
etween FAZA uptake and levels of plasma hepa-
Icyte growth factor, which is an hypoxia-induced
ecreted protein that regulates interleukin-8
xpression.[51] There is clearly a need for compara-
ve studies among FAZA, FMISO, and Cu-ATSM
I determine the optimal hypoxia tracer.

TUMOR PROLIFERATION

One of the most promising areas of research in
HNSCC imaging is the evaluation of cellular proliferation. Chemoradiation therapy has been shown
to reduce proliferation rates in early responding
tumors.[52] Furthermore, this biologic response
typically occurs before reduction in tumor size,
and it is thought that imaging proliferation may
help predict the treatment outcome earlier than
with conventional modalities.[53] Early evaluation
of treatment response may help determine
whether treatment should be modified for more
aggressive management or possibly discontinua-
tion. The most widely studied tumor proliferation
marker for PET is FLT.

FLT

FLT is a nucleoside derivative that is retained in the
cell by thymidine kinase (TK)-1. The enzymatic
activity of TK-1 is increased during the S-phase
of cell cycle. Therefore, FLT uptake in the tissue
is considered a marker of cellular proliferation
although FLT is not incorporated into the DNA.[53]

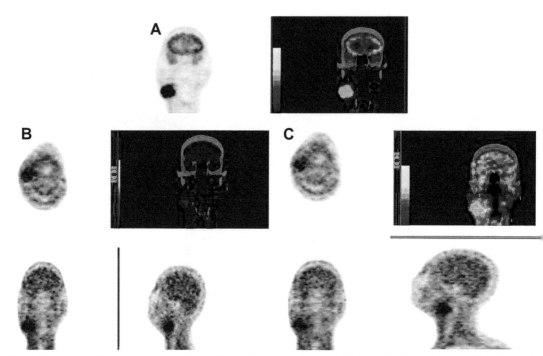

Fig. 2. Examples of typical patient of 3 baseline PET scans performed: (*A*) FDG PET/CT at day 0, (*B*) first FMISO PE scan at day 1, and (*C*) second pretreatment FMISO PET scan at day 4. Note the general similarity of hypoxia trace distribution between 2 pretreatment FMISO PET/CT scans. (*From* Lee N, Nehmeh S, Schoder H, et al. Prospectiv trial incorporating pre-/mid-treatment [18F]-misonidazole positron emission tomography for head-and-nec cancer patients undergoing concurrent chemoradiotherapy. Int J Radiat Oncol Biol Phys 2009;75:101–8; wit permission.)

HNSCCs and their metastases are positively imaged with FLT PET scans. However, in preth-erapy detection of HNSCC, FLT does not seem to offer any advantage compared with FDG.[54,55] FLT uptake also does not seem to be specific to tumor in cervical lymph nodes. Similar FLT uptake was seen in metastatic and reactive nodes in patients with HNSCC.[56] FLT uptake in reactive no-des may be due to proliferation of reactive B-lymphocytes.[56]

The potential role of FLT PET in head and neck cancer will be in the early assessment and moni-toring of treatment response. A study by de Langen and colleagues[57] showed excellent reproducibility of quantitative FLT measurements for tumor prolif-eration, including patients with HNSCC, which is a prerequisite to use this agent as a marker of treatment response. Menda and colleagues[58] examined the kinetic behavior of FLT before and after 10 Gy of radiation therapy combined with chemotherapy. There is a significant decrease in tumor uptake of FLT after 10 Gy of radiation therapy and 1 cycle of chemotherapy (**Fig. 5**). Similar drop in FLT uptake early into radiation therapy was also reported by Troost and colleagues[59] with changes in FLT uptake preceding changes in CT-based tumor volume. There is also near complete

disappearance of FLT uptake in irradiated cervica bone marrow after 10 Gy of radiation therapy, re flecting the drop in cellular proliferation of hematc poietically active tissue. Large clinical trials ar clearly needed to define the role of FLT PET in th management and treatment monitoring of hea and neck cancers.

AMINO ACID METABOLISM

Tumor cells are known to have high nutritiona demands for glucose, amino acids (AAs), an other nutrients. AAs play a key role in cance progression, not only for protein synthesis bu also as a source of carbon and nitrogen for th synthesis of other bioactive molecules.[60,61] I addition to the anabolic need for AAs, malignar tumors have upregulation of AA transport.[60] Regu lation of AA transport is modulated by multipl factors, including hormones, cytokines, and othe mediators. Studies have shown that the expres sion of various transporters correlates with cance progression.[60] Because of the importance of AA in tumor cell function, radiolabeled AA analog may play an important role in identifying tumor bio logic behavior and imaging properties. Recen advancements have been made in terms c

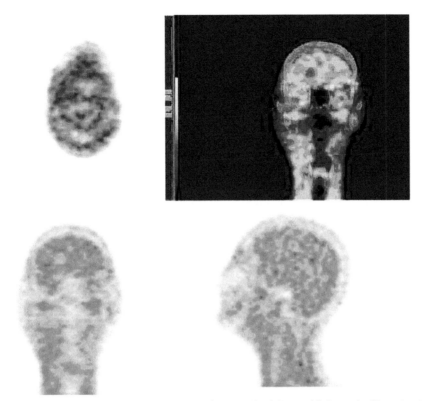

Fig. 3. Example of mid-treatment F-MISO PET/CT scan with no residual detectable hypoxia. (*From* Lee N, Nehmeh S, Schoder H, et al. Prospective trial incorporating pre-/mid-treatment [18F]-misonidazole positron emission tomography for head-and-neck cancer patients undergoing concurrent chemoradiotherapy. Int J Radiat Oncol Biol Phys 2009;75:101–8; with permission.)

imaging of AA metabolism in HNSCC. Radiolabeled AA analogs such as ^{11}C-methionine (C-MET), O-2-fluoro-(^{18}F)-ethyl-L-tyrosine (FET), and L-3-(^{18}F)-fluoro-α-methyltyrosine (FMT) have been developed as PET ligands for tumor detection and have been applied in HNSCC.[62–66]

C-MET

C-MET is one of the most widely used AA tracers. It was first discovered in 1976 by Comar and colleagues,[67,68] and early work in cancer imaging was performed in pancreatic carcinoma. Since then, C-MET has been used for multiple malignancies including HNSCC.[69–76] Early studies using C-MET in head and neck cancer by Leskinen-Kallio and colleagues[63] showed that head and neck cancers of varying histology can be imaged with C-MET.

The role of C-MET, similarly to FLT, may potentially be early evaluation of treatment response. Lindholm and colleagues reported one of the first studies of the use of C-MET in assessing treatment response in head and neck cancers. Fifteen patients, of whom most who had HNSCC,

underwent preradiation and postradiation C-MET scanning. The high C-MET uptake suggested the presence of persistent disease and the marked decrease in C-MET uptake correlated with treatment response. In a similar study, Chesnay and colleagues[77] performed C-MET scanning on 13 patients with locally advanced hypopharyngeal cancer before and after 1 cycle of chemotherapy. They reported that C-MET provided early useful information about changes in tumor metabolism after treatment.

C-MET for tumor delineation in HNSCC has been evaluated and does not seem to provide benefit compared with FDG. Geets and colleagues[78] compared the effectiveness of C-MET, FDG, and CT for delineation of tumor volume in pharyngolaryngeal squamous cell carcinoma. Twenty-three patients with HNSCC were treated with primary radiotherapy or total laryngectomy. CT, FDG, and C-MET images were acquired, and tumor volumes were delineated on CT using an adaptive threshold-based automatic method on FDG and C-MET. Results from their study showed that FDG resulted in a significant reduction of gross target volume compared with CT, while

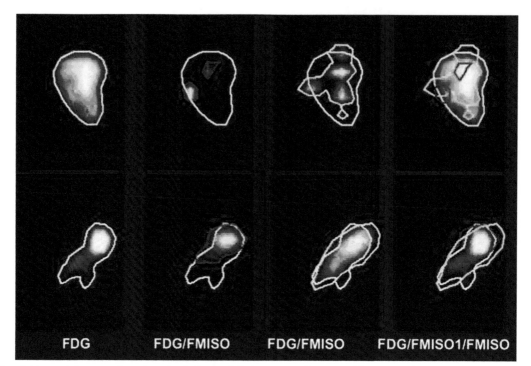

FDG FDG/FMISO FDG/FMISO FDG/FMISO1/FMISO

Fig. 4. Transaxial, coronal, and sagittal views of FDG target volume, and hypoxic volumes in first FMISO an second FMISO as defined by tumor-to-blood (TB) ratio of ≥1.2. Large variability between patients' repeat FMISO scans illustrated for patient with poorest (*top*) and best (*bottom*) correlation between FMISO1 and FMISO2. Images show transaxial, coronal, and sagittal views. (*From* Nehmeh SA, Lee NY, Schroder H, et al. Reproducibilit of intratumor distribution of (18)F-fluoromisonidazole in head and neck cancer. Int J Radiat Oncol Biol Phy 2008;70:235–42; with permission.)

gross tumor volume delineated with C-MET did not differ from CT volumes. While C-MET appears to be promising as a tracer for assessing HNSCC treatment response, further studies are needed establish that role.

FET

FET has been predominantly studied in brain malignancies but its role in HNSCC is under investigation. Early clinical studies of FET showed high in vivo stability and high blood–brain barrier penetration.[79]

Three studies have compared FET and FDG in HNSCC. Pauleit and colleagues[66] compared FET to FDG in 21 patients with head and neck cancers. All patients underwent FDG and FET before treatment. They reported that FDG had a sensitivity of 93%, a specificity of 79%, and an accuracy of 83%, whereas FET had a lower sensitivity of 75% but a higher specificity of 95% and an accuracy of 90%. In a similar study, Balogova and colleagues[80] examined 27 patients with HNSCC comparing FDG and FET. On a per-patient basis, FDG had a sensitivity of 100%, a specificity of 71%, and an accuracy of 93%, whereas FET had

a sensitivity of 70%, a specificity of 100%, an an accuracy of 78%. A recent study by Haerl and colleagues[81] showed that FDG had a sensi tivity of 85%, a specificity of 50%, and an accu racy of 81%, whereas FET had a sensitivity c 70%, a specificity of 90%, and an accuracy c 74%. These studies show that FET cannot replac FDG for the evaluation of HNSCC but may hel differentiate tumor from inflammation.

FMT

FMT was first developed in 1997 by Tomiyoshi anc colleagues.[82] Preclinical studies showed that FMT had rapid blood clearance and maximum tissu uptake in the kidneys and pancreas, similar tc other known AA analogs. Furthermore, FMT demonstrated tumor detectability in nude mic bearing LS180 human colorectal cancer RPM11788 human B-cell lymphoma, and MCF human breast cancer cells, supporting its use as a radiotracer.[83] Since then, FMT has been usec in clinical studies for various cancers.[84–87] Initia studies in head and neck cancers were performec in patients with maxillofacial cancers. Pretreat ment FMT and FDG scans were performed on 30

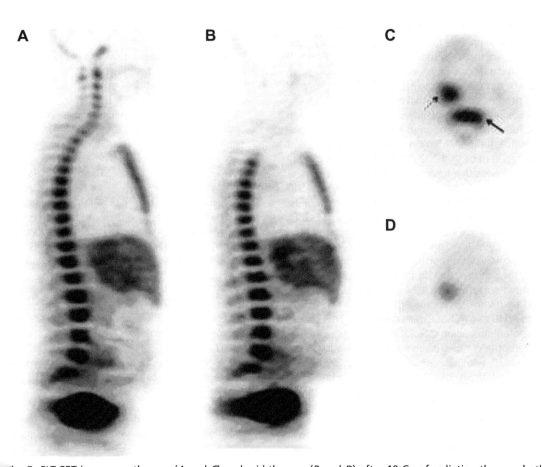

Fig. 5. FLT PET images pretherapy (*A* and *C*) and mid-therapy (*B* and *D*) after 10 Gy of radiation therapy, both obtained at approximately 75 minutes after the intravenous administration of 181 MBq of FLT. Note the disappearance of FLT uptake in the cervical spine and upper thoracic spine on sagittal images (*A* and *B*). Representative transaxial images (*C* and *D*) also show the drop in FLT uptake in the bone marrow (*arrow*) and right tonsillar squamous cell carcinoma (*dashed arrow*) after therapy. (*From* Menda Y, Ponto LL, Dornfeld KJ, et al. Investigation of the pharmacokinetics of 3′-deoxy-3′-[18F]fluorothymidine uptake in the bone marrow before and early after initiation of chemoradiation therapy in head and neck cancer. Nucl Med Biol 2010;37:433–8; with permission.)

patients, with most having squamous cell carcinoma.[65] Results from the study showed that although the differential diagnosis of FMT based on uptake in maxillofacial tumors was no different than that of FDG, FMT had greater contrast than FDG between tumors and surrounding normal structures. More recent studies comparing FMT and FDG were also performed on patients with oral squamous cell carcinoma in whom FMT showed a better correlation to cellular proliferation than that of FDG.[86] There is not enough data to determine the role of FMT, but these early results suggest FMT may provide additional diagnostic information in addition to FDG.

EGFR

EGFR is a well-known receptor TK that is involved in various cellular processes, including proliferation, invasion, induction of angiogenesis, and inhibition of apoptosis.[88,89] Many signaling pathways are involved in EGFR, including Ras-mitogen-activated protein kinase, phosphatidylinositol 3-kinase-phosphatase and tensin homolog-protein kinase B, and phospholipase C pathways.[90] In 1986, Ozanne and colleagues[91] first showed that EGFR overexpression correlated with HNSCC. This was later validated by other studies, leading to therapies targeting EGFR.[92] Two extensively studied strategies for blocking EGFR are the monoclonal antibodies and the low molecular weight TK inhibitors (TKIs).[88] EGFR TKIs bind intracellularly to EGFR TK and inhibit downstream signaling pathways. Currently, the main clinically investigated TKIs are erlotinib and gefitinib.

TKI and EGFR Biomarker Tracers

Erlotinib and gefitinib are 2 TKIs that are widely studied in HNSCC. They act on EGFR by competing with adenosine triphosphate for adenosine triphosphate binding, thus inhibiting autophosphorylation and downstream signal transduction.[62] Phase I and phase II trials using erlotinib for HNSCC have shown modest improvement in overall survival and progression-free survival.[93]

Radiolabeled erlotinib, ^{11}C-labeled erlotinib (^{11}C-erlotinib), has been used to identify erlotinib-sensitive tumors. Memon and colleagues[94] first showed in mice that ^{11}C-erlotinib PET can identify erlotinib-sensitive tumors. In their experiments, 3 human lung cancer cell lines were chosen: A549 and NCI358 expressed low levels of EGFR, whereas HCC827 expressed high levels of EGFR. Human lung cancer cells were xenografted into female BALB/cA nude mice, and micro-PET imaging was performed using ^{11}C-erlotinib. Results from their study showed that xenografts from the erlotinib-sensitive HCC827 cells could be visualized by micro-PET scanning, whereas xenografts from A549 and NCI358 cells could not. This shows the potential of using radiolabeled erlotinib as a tool to detect erlotinib-sensitive tumors. In addition to using ^{11}C-erlotinib, similar imaging strategies were performed by Meng and colleagues[95] in which ^{11}C-labeled 4-N-(3-bromoanilino)-6,7-dimethoxyquinazoline (^{11}C-PD153035), an imaging biomarker of EGFR, was used to detect EGFR TKI-sensitive tumors in patients with non–small cell lung cancer. This study showed a strong correlation between uptake of ^{11}C-PD153035 in the tumor and improved survival of lung cancer patients receiving erlotinib after they have failed chemotherapy. These results suggests that usage of EGFR targeting molecular tracers may be a useful strategy for identifying head and neck cancers that are susceptible to EGFR target treatment.

SUMMARY

New PET tracers allow the evaluation of important biologic characteristics of HNSCC, including hypoxia, cell proliferation, and drug susceptibility. These radiopharmaceuticals are expected to complement FDG to allow better understanding of the biologic profiles of the tumors, leading potentially to more personalized therapies. The experience with these agents in human cancer imaging is variable. Although FLT and FMISO have been more extensively investigated than others, larger clinical trials are needed to determine the clinical role of these radiopharmaceuticals in HNSCC.

REFERENCES

1. Fischbein NJ, OS AA, Caputo GR, et al. Clinical utility of positron emission tomography with 18F-fluorodeoxyglucose in detecting residual/recurrent squamous cell carcinoma of the head and neck. AJNR Am J Neuroradiol 1998;19:1189–96.

2. Krabbe CA, Pruim J, van der Laan BF, et al. FDG-PET and detection of distant metastases and simultaneous tumors in head and neck squamous cell carcinoma: a comparison with chest radiography and chest CT. Oral Oncol 2009;45:234–40.

3. Lapela M, Grenman R, Kurki T, et al. Head and neck cancer: detection of recurrence with PET and 2-[F-18]fluoro-2-deoxy-D-glucose. Radiology 1995;197: 205–11.

4. Ng SH, Chan SC, Liao CT, et al. Distant metastases and synchronous second primary tumors in patients with newly diagnosed oropharyngeal and hypopharyngeal carcinomas: evaluation of (18)F-FDG PET and extended-field multi-detector row CT. Neuroradiology 2008;50:969–79.

5. Senft A, de Bree R, Hoekstra OS, et al. Screening for distant metastases in head and neck cancer patients by chest CT or whole body FDG-PET: a prospective multicenter trial. Radiother Oncol 2008;87:221–9.

6. Becker A, Hansgen G, Bloching M, et al. Oxygenation of squamous cell carcinoma of the head and neck: comparison of primary tumors, neck node metastases, and normal tissue. Int J Radiat Oncol Biol Phys 1998;42:35–41.

7. Brizel DM, Sibley GS, Prosnitz LR, et al. Tumor hypoxia adversely affects the prognosis of carcinoma of the head and neck. Int J Radiat Oncol Biol Phys 1997;38:285–9.

8. Nordsmark M, Bentzen SM, Rudat V, et al. Prognostic value of tumor oxygenation in 397 head and neck tumors after primary radiation therapy. An international multi-center study. Radiother Oncol 2005; 77:18–24.

9. Bristow RG, Hill RP. Hypoxia and metabolism. Hypoxia, DNA repair and genetic instability. Nat Rev Cancer 2008;8:180–92.

10. Schoder H, Fury M, Lee N, et al. PET monitoring of therapy response in head and neck squamous cell carcinoma. J Nucl Med 2009;50(Suppl 1):74S–88S.

11. Corry J, Rischin D. Strategies to overcome accelerated repopulation and hypoxia: what have we learned from clinical trials? Semin Oncol 2004;31: 802–8.

12. Erler JT, Cawthorne CJ, Williams KJ, et al. Hypoxia-mediated down-regulation of Bid and Bax in tumors occurs via hypoxia-inducible factor 1-dependent and -independent mechanisms and contributes to drug resistance. Mol Cell Biol 2004;24:2875–89.

13. Gerweck LE, Kozin SV, Stocks SJ. The pH partition theory predicts the accumulation and toxicity of doxorubicin in normal and low-pH-adapted cells. Br J Cancer 1999;79:838–42.

4. Kyle AH, Huxham LA, Yeoman DM, et al. Limited tissue penetration of taxanes: a mechanism for resistance in solid tumors. Clin Cancer Res 2007;13: 2804–10.

5. Teicher BA, Lazo JS, Sartorelli AC. Classification of antineoplastic agents by their selective toxicities toward oxygenated and hypoxic tumor cells. Cancer Res 1981;41:73–81.

6. Wilson WR, Hay MP. Targeting hypoxia in cancer therapy. Nat Rev Cancer 2011;11:393–410.

7. Yoshiba S, Ito D, Nagumo T, et al. Hypoxia induces resistance to 5-fluorouracil in oral cancer cells via G(1) phase cell cycle arrest. Oral Oncol 2009;45: 109–15.

8. Schoder H, Ong SC. Fundamentals of molecular imaging: rationale and applications with relevance for radiation oncology. Semin Nucl Med 2008;38: 119–28.

9. Tatum JL, Kelloff GJ, Gillies RJ, et al. Hypoxia: importance in tumor biology, noninvasive measurement by imaging, and value of its measurement in the management of cancer therapy. Int J Radiat Biol 2006;82:699–757.

10. Eschmann SM, Paulsen F, Reimold M, et al. Prognostic impact of hypoxia imaging with 18F-misonidazole PET in non-small cell lung cancer and head and neck cancer before radiotherapy. J Nucl Med 2005; 46:253–60.

11. Troost EG, Schinagl DA, Bussink J, et al. Innovations in radiotherapy planning of head and neck cancers: role of PET. J Nucl Med 2009;51:66–76.

12. Graham MM, Peterson LM, Link JM, et al. Fluorine-18-fluoromisonidazole radiation dosimetry in imaging studies. J Nucl Med 1997;38:1631–6.

13. Hendrickson K, Phillips M, Smith W, et al. Hypoxia imaging with [F-18] FMISO-PET in head and neck cancer: potential for guiding intensity modulated radiation therapy in overcoming hypoxia-induced treatment resistance. Radiother Oncol 2011;101:369–75.

14. Koh WJ, Rasey JS, Evans ML, et al. Imaging of hypoxia in human tumors with [F-18]fluoromisonidazole. Int J Radiat Oncol Biol Phys 1992;22:199–212.

15. Rajendran JG, Schwartz DL, O'Sullivan J, et al. Tumor hypoxia imaging with [F-18] fluoromisonidazole positron emission tomography in head and neck cancer. Clin Cancer Res 2006;12:5435–41.

16. Rasey JS, Koh WJ, Grierson JR, et al. Radiolabelled fluoromisonidazole as an imaging agent for tumor hypoxia. Int J Radiat Oncol Biol Phys 1989; 17:985–91.

17. Wen B, Burgman P, Zanzonico P, et al. A preclinical model for noninvasive imaging of hypoxia-induced gene expression; comparison with an exogenous marker of tumor hypoxia. Eur J Nucl Med Mol Imaging 2004;31:1530–8.

28. Srinivasan A, Mohan S, Mukherji SK. Biologic imaging of head and neck cancer: the present and the future. AJNR Am J Neuroradiol 2011;33(4): 586–94.

29. Gagel B, Reinartz P, Dimartino E, et al. pO(2) Polarography versus positron emission tomography ([(18) F] fluoromisonidazole, [(18)F]-2-fluoro-2'-deoxyglucose). An appraisal of radiotherapeutically relevant hypoxia. Strahlenther Onkol 2004;180:616–22.

30. Hicks RJ, Rischin D, Fisher R, et al. Utility of FMISO PET in advanced head and neck cancer treated with chemoradiation incorporating a hypoxia-targeting chemotherapy agent. Eur J Nucl Med Mol Imaging 2005;32:1384–91.

31. Jansen JF, Schoder H, Lee NY, et al. Noninvasive assessment of tumor microenvironment using dynamic contrast-enhanced magnetic resonance imaging and 18F-fluoromisonidazole positron emission tomography imaging in neck nodal metastases. Int J Radiat Oncol Biol Phys 2010;77:1403–10.

32. Lee N, Nehmeh S, Schoder H, et al. Prospective trial incorporating pre-/mid-treatment [18F]-misonidazole positron emission tomography for head-and-neck cancer patients undergoing concurrent chemoradiotherapy. Int J Radiat Oncol Biol Phys 2009;75:101–8.

33. Lee NY, Mechalakos JG, Nehmeh S, et al. Fluorine-18-labeled fluoromisonidazole positron emission and computed tomography-guided intensity-modulated radiotherapy for head and neck cancer: a feasibility study. Int J Radiat Oncol Biol Phys 2008;70:2–13.

34. Nehmeh SA, Lee NY, Schroder H, et al. Reproducibility of intratumor distribution of (18)F-fluoromisonidazole in head and neck cancer. Int J Radiat Oncol Biol Phys 2008;70:235–42.

35. Rischin D, Hicks RJ, Fisher R, et al. Prognostic significance of [18F]-misonidazole positron emission tomography-detected tumor hypoxia in patients with advanced head and neck cancer randomly assigned to chemoradiation with or without tirapazamine: a substudy of Trans-Tasman Radiation Oncology Group Study 98.02. J Clin Oncol 2006; 24:2098–104.

36. Thorwarth D, Eschmann SM, Holzner F, et al. Combined uptake of [18F]FDG and [18F]FMISO correlates with radiation therapy outcome in head-and-neck cancer patients. Radiother Oncol 2006; 80:151–6.

37. Thorwarth D, Eschmann SM, Paulsen F, et al. A kinetic model for dynamic [18F]-Fmiso PET data to analyse tumour hypoxia. Phys Med Biol 2005;50: 2209–24.

38. Wang W, Lee NY, Georgi JC, et al. Pharmacokinetic analysis of hypoxia (18)F-fluoromisonidazole dynamic PET in head and neck cancer. J Nucl Med 2010;51:37–45.

39. Rasey JS, Koh WJ, Evans ML, et al. Quantifying regional hypoxia in human tumors with positron

emission tomography of [18F]fluoromisonidazole: a pretherapy study of 37 patients. Int J Radiat Oncol Biol Phys 1996;36:417–28.

40. Hong YT, Beech JS, Smith R, et al. Parametric mapping of [18F]fluoromisonidazole positron emission tomography using basis functions. J Cereb Blood Flow Metab 2011;31:648–57.

41. Wang W, Georgi JC, Nehmeh SA, et al. Evaluation of a compartmental model for estimating tumor hypoxia via FMISO dynamic PET imaging. Phys Med Biol 2009;54:3083–99.

42. Eschmann SM, Paulsen F, Bedeshem C, et al. Hypoxia-imaging with (18)F-misonidazole and PET: changes of kinetics during radiotherapy of head-and-neck cancer. Radiother Oncol 2007;83:406–10.

43. Holland JP, Lewis JS, Dehdashti F. Assessing tumor hypoxia by positron emission tomography with Cu-ATSM. Q J Nucl Med Mol Imaging 2009;53:193–200.

44. Dearling JL, Packard AB. Some thoughts on the mechanism of cellular trapping of Cu(II)-ATSM. Nucl Med Biol 2010;37:237–43.

45. Chao KS, Bosch WR, Mutic S, et al. A novel approach to overcome hypoxic tumor resistance: Cu-ATSM-guided intensity-modulated radiation therapy. Int J Radiat Oncol Biol Phys 2001;49: 1171–82.

46. Kositwattanarerk A, Oh M, Kudo T, et al. Different distribution of (2)Cu ATSM and (1)F-FDG in head and neck cancers. Clin Nucl Med 2012;37:252–7.

47. Minagawa Y, Shizukuishi K, Koike I, et al. Assessment of tumor hypoxia by 62Cu-ATSM PET/CT as a predictor of response in head and neck cancer: a pilot study. Ann Nucl Med 2011;25:339–45.

48. Piert M, Machulla HJ, Picchio M, et al. Hypoxia-specific tumor imaging with 18F-fluoroazomycin arabinoside. J Nucl Med 2005;46:106–13.

49. Grosu AL, Souvatzoglou M, Roper B, et al. Hypoxia imaging with FAZA-PET and theoretical considerations with regard to dose painting for individualization of radiotherapy in patients with head and neck cancer. Int J Radiat Oncol Biol Phys 2007;69:541–51.

50. Souvatzoglou M, Grosu AL, Roper B, et al. Tumour hypoxia imaging with [18F]FAZA PET in head and neck cancer patients: a pilot study. Eur J Nucl Med Mol Imaging 2007;34:1566–75.

51. Le QT, Fisher R, Oliner KS, et al. Prognostic and predictive significance of plasma HGF and IL-8 in a phase III trial of chemoradiation with or without tirapazamine in locoregionally advanced head and neck cancer. Clin Cancer Res 2012;18:1798–807.

52. Weber WA. Monitoring tumor response to therapy with 18F-FLT PET. J Nucl Med 2010;51:841–4.

53. Bading JR, Shields AF. Imaging of cell proliferation: status and prospects. J Nucl Med 2008;49(Suppl 2): 64S–80S.

54. Hoshikawa H, Nishiyama Y, Kishino T, et al. Comparison of FLT-PET and FDG-PET for visualization of

55. Cobben DC, van der Laan BF, Maas B, et al. 18F-FL PET for visualization of laryngeal cancer: compariso with 18F-FDG PET. J Nucl Med 2004;45:226–31.

56. Troost EG, Vogel WV, Merkx MA, et al. 18F-FLT PE does not discriminate between reactive and meta static lymph nodes in primary head and neck canc patients. J Nucl Med 2007;48:726–35.

57. de Langen AJ, Klabbers B, Lubberink M, et a Reproducibility of quantitative 18F-3'-deoxy-3'-fluo rothymidine measurements using positron emissic tomography. Eur J Nucl Med Mol Imaging 2009;3 389–95.

58. Menda Y, Boles Ponto LL, Dornfeld KJ, et al. Kinet analysis of 3'-deoxy-3'-(18)F-fluorothymidine ((18) FLT) in head and neck cancer patients before ar early after initiation of chemoradiation therap J Nucl Med 2009;50:1028–35.

59. Troost EG, Bussink J, Hoffmann AL, et al. 18F-FL PET/CT for early response monitoring and dos escalation in oropharyngeal tumors. J Nucl Me 2010;51:866–74.

60. Haberkorn U, Markert A, Mier W, et al. Molecula imaging of tumor metabolism and apoptosis. Onco gene 2011;30:4141–51.

61. Kaira K, Oriuchi N, Sunaga N, et al. A system review of PET and biology in lung cancer. Am Transl Res 2011;3:383–91.

62. Heuveling DA, de Bree R, van Dongen GA. Th potential role of non-FDG-PET in the managemer of head and neck cancer. Oral Oncol 2011;47:2–7

63. Leskinen-Kallio S, Nagren K, Lehikoinen P, et a Carbon-11-methionine and PET is an effectiv method to image head and neck cancer. J Nuc Med 1992;33:691–5.

64. Lindholm P, Leskinen S, Lapela M. Carbon-11-meth onine uptake in squamous cell head and nec cancer. J Nucl Med 1998;39:1393–7.

65. Miyakubo M, Oriuchi N, Tsushima Y, et al. Diagnosi of maxillofacial tumor with L-3-[18F]-fluoro-alpha methyltyrosine (FMT) PET: a comparative stud with FDG-PET. Ann Nucl Med 2007;21:129–35.

66. Pauleit D, Zimmermann A, Stoffels G, et al. 18F-FE PET compared with 18F-FDG PET and CT in patien with head and neck cancer. J Nucl Med 2006;47 256–61.

67. Comar D, Cartron J, Maziere M, et al. Labelling an metabolism of methionine-methyl-11 C. Eur J Nuc Med 1976;1:11–4.

68. Syrota A, Comar D, Cerf M, et al. [11C]Methionin pancreatic scanning with positron emissio computed tomography. J Nucl Med 1979;20:778–81

69. Leskinen-Kallio S, Minn H, Joensuu H. PET an [11C]methionine in assessment of respons in non-Hodgkin lymphoma. Lancet 1990;336 1188.

). Leskinen-Kallio S, Ruotsalainen U, Nagren K, et al. Uptake of carbon-11-methionine and fluorodeoxyglucose in non-Hodgkin's lymphoma: a PET study. J Nucl Med 1991;32:1211–8.

. Lindholm P, Lapela M, Nagren K, et al. Preliminary study of carbon-11 methionine PET in the evaluation of early response to therapy in advanced breast cancer. Nucl Med Commun 2009;30:30–6.

2. Lindholm P, Leskinen S, Nagren K, et al. Carbon-11-methionine PET imaging of malignant melanoma. J Nucl Med 1995;36:1806–10.

3. Sasaki M, Kuwabara Y, Yoshida T, et al. Comparison of MET-PET and FDG-PET for differentiation between benign lesions and malignant tumors of the lung. Ann Nucl Med 2001;15:425–31.

4. Singhal T, Narayanan TK, Jain V, et al. 11C-L-Methionine positron emission tomography in the clinical management of cerebral gliomas. Mol Imaging Biol 2008;10:1–18.

5. Wieder H, Ott K, Zimmermann F, et al. PET imaging with [11C]methyl- L-methionine for therapy monitoring in patients with rectal cancer. Eur J Nucl Med Mol Imaging 2002;29:789–96.

6. Wong TZ, van der Westhuizen GJ, Coleman RE. Positron emission tomography imaging of brain tumors. Neuroimaging Clin N Am 2002;12:615–26.

7. Chesnay E, Babin E, Constans JM, et al. Early response to chemotherapy in hypopharyngeal cancer: assessment with (11)C-methionine PET, correlation with morphologic response, and clinical outcome. J Nucl Med 2003;44:526–32.

8. Geets X, Daisne JF, Gregoire V, et al. Role of 11-C-methionine positron emission tomography for the delineation of the tumor volume in pharyngolaryngeal squamous cell carcinoma: comparison with FDG-PET and CT. Radiother Oncol 2004;71:267–73.

9. Wester HJ, Herz M, Weber W, et al. Synthesis and radiopharmacology of O-(2-[18F]fluoroethyl)-L-tyrosine for tumor imaging. J Nucl Med 1999;40:205–12.

0. Balogova S, Perie S, Kerrou K, et al. Prospective comparison of FDG and FET PET/CT in patients with head and neck squamous cell carcinoma. Mol Imaging Biol 2008;10:364–73.

1. Haerle SK, Fischer DR, Schmid DT, et al. 18F-FET PET/CT in advanced head and neck squamous cell carcinoma: an intra-individual comparison with 18F-FDG PET/CT. Mol Imaging Biol 2011;13:1036–42.

2. Tomiyoshi K, Amed K, Muhammad S, et al. Synthesis of isomers of 18F-labelled amino acid radiopharmaceutical: position 2- and 3-L-18F-alpha-methyltyrosine using a separation and purification system. Nucl Med Commun 1997;18:169–75.

83. Inoue T, Tomiyoshi K, Higuichi T, et al. Biodistributionstudies on L-3-[fluorine-18]fluoro-alpha-methyl tyrosine: a potential tumor-detecting agent. J Nucl Med 1998;39:663–7.

84. Kaira K, Oriuchi N, Otani Y, et al. Fluorine-18-alpha-methyltyrosine positron emission tomography for diagnosis and staging of lung cancer: a clinicopathologic study. Clin Cancer Res 2007;13:6369–78.

85. Kaira K, Oriuchi N, Shimizu K, et al. Evaluation of thoracic tumors with (18)F-FMT and (18)F-FDG PET-CT: a clinicopathological study. Int J Cancer 2009;124:1152–60.

86. Miyashita G, Higuchi T, Oriuchi N, et al. 18F-FAMT uptake correlates with tumor proliferative activity in oral squamous cell carcinoma: comparative study with 18F-FDG PET and immunohistochemistry. Ann Nucl Med 2010;24:579–84.

87. Sohda M, Kato H, Suzuki S, et al. 18F-FAMT-PET is useful for the diagnosis of lymph node metastasis in operable esophageal squamous cell carcinoma. Ann Surg Oncol 2010;17:3181–6.

88. Gold KA, Lee HY, Kim ES. Targeted therapies in squamous cell carcinoma of the head and neck. Cancer 2009;115:922–35.

89. Sharafinski ME, Ferris RL, Ferrone S, et al. Epidermal growth factor receptor targeted therapy of squamous cell carcinoma of the head and neck. Head Neck 2010;32:1412–21.

90. Hynes NE, Lane HA. ERBB receptors and cancer: the complexity of targeted inhibitors. Nat Rev Cancer 2005;5:341–54.

91. Ozanne B, Richards CS, Hendler F, et al. Overexpression of the EGF receptor is a hallmark of squamous cell carcinomas. J Pathol 1986;149:9–14.

92. Leemans CR, Braakhuis BJ, Brakenhoff RH. The molecular biology of head and neck cancer. Nat Rev Cancer 2011;11:9–22.

93. Soulieres D, Senzer NN, Vokes EE, et al. Multicenter phase II study of erlotinib, an oral epidermal growth factor receptor tyrosine kinase inhibitor, in patients with recurrent or metastatic squamous cell cancer of the head and neck. J Clin Oncol 2004; 22:77–85.

94. Memon AA, Jakobsen S, Dagnaes-Hansen F, et al. Positron emission tomography (PET) imaging with [11C]-labeled erlotinib: a micro-PET study on mice with lung tumor xenografts. Cancer Res 2009;69: 873–8.

95. Meng X, Loo BW Jr, Ma L, et al. Molecular imaging with 11C-PD153035 PET/CT predicts survival in non-small cell lung cancer treated with EGFR-TKI: a pilot study. J Nucl Med 2011;52:1573–9.

Positron Emission Tomography in Head and Neck Squamous Cell Carcinoma of Unknown Primary

Kimberly J. Kinder, MD[a], Pierre Lavertu, MD[a],*,
Min Yao, MD, PhD[b]

KEYWORDS

- FDG-PET • Carcinoma of unknown primary • Head and neck squamous cell carcinoma • Workup

KEY POINTS

- FDG-PET is a useful imaging modality in the workup of head and neck carcinoma of unknown primary, allowing detection of an occult primary tumor that may be missed by a conventional workup.
- In some situations, it is helpful to obtain FDG-PET before panendoscopy and biopsies. The decision of when to obtain a PET scan should be made by the multidisciplinary treatment team.
- One should be careful in interpreting PET results because of considerably high false-positive rates and false-negative rates.
- Owing to the current limitations of PET imaging, routine panendoscopy with biopsies should still be performed for patients with negative PET studies.

INTRODUCTION

Carcinoma of unknown primary (CUP) is 1 of the 10 most common cancers, representing 3% to 5% of all malignancies.[1] Prognosis is generally poor, with reported average survival of only 6 to 10 months.[2] The primary tumor is identified in fewer than 20% of patients, even with an extensive workup, and only in 70% of autopsy studies.[3] When a primary site is eventually identified in the patient initially diagnosed as CUP, the most common primary sites are lung, oropharynx, nasopharynx, breast, colorectal area, and esophagus, in descending order.[4]

Cervical metastases with an unknown primary (HNCUP for head and neck carcinoma of unknown primary) make up anywhere from one-quarter to two-thirds of all CUP cases.[4,5] Patients with HNCUP tend to do much better than patients with lymphadenopathy at other sites, with an average 5-year survival of 35% to 50%.[6,7] In patients with HNCUP, the primary tumor is detected in fewer than 40% of patients with workup, and in 80% of patients at autopsy.[8] Identification of a primary site permits the clinician to tailor the therapy to address only the involved area. This allows for potential surgical treatment of disease, as well as modification of the radiation fields and thus potential reduction of radiation side effects. This article reviews the relevant anatomy and conventional workup in patients with HNCUP and discusses the use of positron emission tomography (PET) imaging in this population.

ANATOMY

Head and neck cancer comprises only about 2% to 4% of cancers in the western hemisphere, but

[a] Department of Otolaryngology–Head and Neck Surgery, University Hospitals Case Medical Center, Case Western Reserve University, 11100 Euclid Avenue, Cleveland, OH 44106, USA; [b] Department of Radiation Oncology, University Hospitals Case Medical Center, Case Western Reserve University, 11100 Euclid Avenue, Cleveland, OH 44106, USA
* Corresponding author.
E-mail address: pierre.lavertu@uhhospitals.org

PET Clin 7 (2012) 443–452
http://dx.doi.org/10.1016/j.cpet.2012.06.007
1556-8598/12/$ – see front matter © 2012 Elsevier Inc. All rights reserved.

Table 1		
Incidence and mortality of head and neck cancer by site, 2010		
Site	Incidence	Deaths
Oral cavity	23,880	5470
Pharynx (includes oropharynx, nasopharynx, and hypopharynx)	12,660	2410
Larynx	12,720	3600

From Jemal A, Siegel R, Xu J, et al. Cancer statistics, 2010. CA Cancer J Clin 2010;60:277–300; with permission.

up to 40% of all malignancies in some Asian countries.[9] The vast majority of head and neck cancers in the western world are squamous cell carcinomas that originate from the lining of the upper aerodigestive tract. The most common sites of head and neck cancer are oral cavity, pharynx, and larynx (**Table 1**).[10]

In contrast to the site-specific incidence in head and neck cancer, the oropharynx is the most common site in HNCUP. This is likely true for several reasons. Oral cavity cancers can be directly visualized and palpated more easily than those in the oropharynx. Tonsillar crypts, which are lined with squamous epithelium, may hide small tumors that cannot be readily seen. The tongue base and associated lingual tonsils have variable folds and protrusions that can be difficult to differentiate from tumor on imaging or clinical examination.

Multiple studies have reported the incidence of primary tumors identified in HNCUP based on anatomic site. In a retrospective study of 23 patients with HNCUP over a 15-year period, primary tumors were eventually identified in 12 patients (53%).[11] The tonsillar fossa harbored 45% of malignancies and an additional 44% were found in the tongue base. Another retrospective study by Wong and colleagues[12] found 14 tongue base tumors and 14 tonsillar tumors in the 30 patients with HNCUP in whom a tumor was identified. In a prospective Korean study, there were 5 tonsillar primaries and 2 primary lesions each in the tongue base and nasopharynx.[13] As one would expect, nasopharyngeal primary tumors are more common in regions with a higher prevalence of Epstein-Barr virus (EBV)-related tumors.[14]

The nodal drainage patterns of the head and neck have been extensively studied, so the location of the involved lymph node helps predict the primary site.[15,16] The neck is divided into lymph node levels by both anatomic and radiographic boundaries (**Fig. 1, Table 2**).[17,18] These divisions

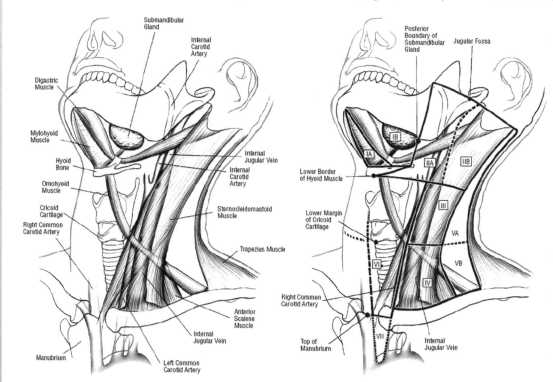

Fig. 1. Diagram of the neck demonstrating relevant anatomy (*left*) and lymph node levels (*right*). (*Reprinted from* Som PM, Curtin HD, Mancuso AA. An imaging-based classification for the cervical nodes designed as an adjunct to recent clinically based nodal classifications. Arch Otolaryngol Head Neck Surg 1999;125:388–96; with permission.

Table 2
Summary of imaging-based nodal classification

Level Number	Nodal Group	Boundaries
Level I	Submental and submandibular nodes	Superior to hyoid bone, inferior to mylohyoid muscle, and anterior to posterior aspect of submandibular gland
Level IA	Submental nodes	Between medial margins of anterior bellies of digastric muscles
Level IB	Submandibular nodes	Lateral to the level IA nodes and anterior to posterior aspect of submandibular gland
Level II	Upper internal jugular nodes	Skull base to inferior border of hyoid bone between posterior aspect of submandibular gland and posterior aspect of sternocleidomastoid muscle
Level IIA		A level II node that lies either anterior, medial, lateral, or posterior to the internal jugular vein. If posterior to the vein, the node is inseparable from the vein.
Level IIB		A level II node that lies posterior to the internal jugular vein and has a fat plane separating it and the vein
Level III	Middle jugular nodes	Between inferior aspect of hyoid bone and inferior border of cricoid arch anterior to posterior border of sternocleidomastoid muscle
Level IV	Low jugular nodes	From inferior border of cricoid arch to clavicle between carotid sheath and sternocleidomastoid muscle
Level V	Posterior triangle nodes	Between posterior border of sternocleidomastoid muscle and anterior border of trapezius muscle from skull base to clavicle
Level VA	Upper level V nodes	Extend from skull base to inferior border of cricoid arch
Level VB	Lower level V nodes	Extend from inferior border of cricoid arch the clavicle
Level VI	Upper visceral nodes	Between the carotid arteries from inferior border of hyoid bone to superior border of manubrium
Level VII	Superior mediastinal nodes	Between the carotid arteries from superior border of manubrium to the level of the innominate vein
No level number	Supraclavicular nodes	At or caudal to the level of the clavicle and lateral to the carotid artery on each side of the neck
No level number	Retropharyngeal nodes	Medial to the internal carotid arteries within 2 cm of the skull base

Adapted from Som PM, Curtin HD, Mancuso AA. An imaging-based classification for the cervical nodes designed as an adjunct to recent clinically based nodal classifications. Arch Otolaryngol Head Neck Surg 1999;125:388–96; with permission.

are helpful both in communicating among clinicians and localizing the primary tumor.

Malignant lymphadenopathy in patients with HNCUP is most commonly seen in level II.[6,19] Level III is the next most frequent region, whereas nodal metastases are seen less often in levels I, IV, and V. Ninety percent of patients have unilateral disease, and 5% to 10% have bilateral lymphadenopathy.[6] **Fig. 2** illustrates the distribution of the involved lymph nodes in 352 consecutive patients with HNCUP seen from 1975 to 1995 in a national survey by the Danish Society for Head and Neck Oncology.[6] Upper and mid-neck metastases usually arise from a head and neck primary. For lower neck and supraclavicular nodes, the primary lesion is usually found below the clavicle. The lung is by far the most common infraclavicular site.[14]

CONVENTIONAL WORKUP

The initial workup for patients with HNCUP consists of a complete history and physical examination in the office. Examination by a trained otolaryngologist includes inspection and, when possible, palpation of the skin, oral cavity, oropharynx, nasopharynx, hypopharynx, larynx, and neck. Most practitioners will use a flexible fiberoptic endoscope, as it allows a detailed examination with minimal patient discomfort.

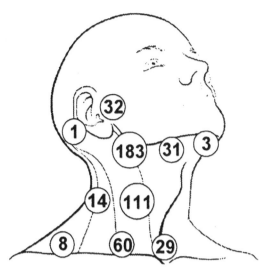

Fig. 2. Involved lymph nodes in 352 HNCUP patients. (*Reprinted from* Grau C, Johansen LV, Jakobsen J, et al. Cervical lymph node metastases from unknown primary tumors. Results from a national survey by the Danish Society for Head and Neck Oncology. Radiother Oncol 2000;55:121–9; with permission.)

In the absence of an obvious primary lesion, tissue should be obtained from the lymph node to confirm malignancy. This is most commonly done via fine-needle aspiration (FNA). Human papillomavirus (HPV) and EBV typing can be performed on tissue obtained via FNA or open biopsy, as this may help to suggest a primary tumor site.[16,20] HPV is most commonly seen in oropharyngeal tumors, whereas many nasopharyngeal tumors are EBV-positive. Identification of the distinct nonkeratinizing morphology seen in HPV-positive tumors is a reliable predictor of a primary source in the oropharynx.[20,21]

If a primary tumor is not found on office examination, imaging studies are recommended. Th should consist of computed tomography (C with contrast or magnetic resonance imagir (MRI) with gadolinium of the head and neck, well as chest radiograph or CT.[22]

After office examination and convention imaging, the primary tumor is identified in mo than 90% of patients. However, these investiga tions fail to reveal a primary lesion in 2% to 8 of cases.[19,23–26] The next step in the workup these patients varies among institutions. Som clinicians will proceed to examination under ane thesia (EUA) with biopsies of clinically suspiciou and clinically probable sites, whereas others w perform PET before EUA. The National Compre hensive Cancer Network (NCCN) currently recom mends PET scan before panendoscopy in thes cases.[22] However, this is a decision that shou be made by the multidisciplinary treatment tea on a case-by-case basis.

PET IMAGING

FDG-PET is a functional imaging modality that use radioactive fluoro-2-deoxy-glucose (FDG) to ider tify metabolically hyperactive cells (**Fig. 3**). Malig nant tissues take up the glucose analog at a highe rate than the normal neighboring cells. Increase FDG-avidity can also be seen in inflammatory an infectious conditions, as well as metabolically activ tissues such as brain, heart, and muscle.

The use of PET in general CUP patients wa initially reported in the early 1990s,[27] and sever published reviews have evaluated the effective ness of PET scans in identifying primary tumors i CUP at multiple body sites.[4,5,8] The reported sens tivity and specificity of PET varied widely. Eac

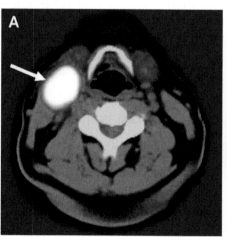
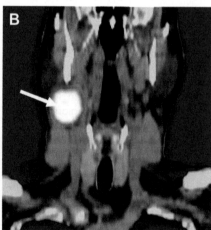

Fig. 3. PET/CT of a patient who presented with an enlarged right level II lymph node (*arrow*) confirmed to hav metastatic squamous cell carcinoma. Extensive workup did not reveal the primary tumor. (*A*) Axial; (*B*) Corona

Table 3
PET characteristics in general cancer of unknown primary syndrome

	Study Type	No. of Patients	Sensitivity (%)	Specificity (%)	Positive Predictive Value (%)	Negative Predictive Value (%)	Tumor Detection Rate (%)
Delgado-Bolton et al[4]	Meta-analysis	298	87	71			43
Freudenberg et al[8]	Literature review	808	47	80	70	93	47
Fencl et al[5]	Retrospective review	451	62	82			47

tudy had its own mix of metastatic foci, histologic ımor types, and data definitions. This review ocuses on squamous cell carcinoma, but many f the studies reported in the literature include ultiple histologic tumor types. Furthermore, ost publications are single institutional retrospective studies containing small patient samples over long period.

Table 3 summarizes representative studies on the use of PET in patients with CUP. One can ee that the addition of PET scan in these patients llows detection of a primary tumor in more than 0% of patients where it could not be found with onventional workup alone.

Results of PET Without Integrated CT in HNCUP

The use of PET limited to HNCUP has been nalyzed in both retrospective and prospective tudies.[25,26,28–34] Rusthoven and colleagues[34] ummarized 16 retrospective studies with a total f 302 patients with HNCUP who had FDG-PET, nd reported that PET had a sensitivity of 88% nd a specificity of 75% in detecting a primary umor. PET detected 24.5% of primary tumors hat were not detected by conventional workup.

The largest prospective study was done by the Danish Head and Neck Cancer Study Group (DA-HANCA-13), which enrolled 60 patients.[30] Patients underwent clinical examination and conventional imaging studies, followed by either PET or PET/CT. PET was not differentiated from PET/CT in reporting the results. The data from this study and 2 additional prospective studies are summarized in Table 4.[29–31] The sensitivity, specificity, positive predictive value, and negative predictive value for detection of a primary tumor from 3 retrospective studies are also shown.[26,28,33]

Results of PET/CT in HNCUP

One of the problems with PET scanning alone is the lack of anatomic detail. In 1998, integrated PET/CT scanners were made available that could perform concurrent full-body PET imaging and CT.[1] This allows PET data to be superimposed on cross-sectional images, which provides much improved anatomic localization.

A recent prospective study reported results of 30 patients with HNCUP who underwent PET/CT.[25] PET/CT was performed after conventional workup and before operative panendoscopy. The surgeons were blinded to the results. Patients had routine

Table 4
PET characteristics in cervical cancer of unknown primary syndrome

	Study Type	No. of Patients	Sensitivity (%)	Specificity (%)	Positive Predictive Value (%)	Negative Predictive Value (%)	Tumor Detection Rate (%)
Johansen et al[30]	Prospective	60	86	69	60	90	29
Silva et al[31]	Prospective	25	60	70	33	87	12
Padovani et al[29]	Prospective	13	70	33	78	25	54
Dandekar et al[28]	Retrospective	59	93	71	56	96	39
Yabuki et al[26]	Retrospective	24	81	77	75	83	37
Wong and Saunders[33]	Retrospective	17	62	66	62	62	47

examination under anesthesia and directed biopsies, and the PET/CT results were then revealed to the surgeon intraoperatively. Additional biopsies were taken if the PET/CT was positive. The traditional workup identified tumors in 25% of patients, whereas PET/CT-directed biopsies revealed the primary lesion in 55% of patients. The sensitivity, specificity, positive predictive value, and negative predictive value of PET/CT in detection of primary tumor were 92%, 63%, 79%, and 83%, respectively.

Hu and colleagues[14] reported a larger Chinese study in 2009. Ninety-three patients underwent PET/CT for HNCUP over a 3-year period. Forty cases were considered definitively positive on PET/CT, and in all of these, the primary sites were confirmed clinically or pathologically. Twenty-eight cases were determined to be "suspicious" on PET/CT, and in 16 (57%) of these, the primary sites were confirmed. However, there were 2 endoscopy-confirmed tumors that were missed on PET/CT.

Wartski and colleagues[35] reviewed 38 consecutive patients who had PET/CT after negative conventional workup including negative EUA. Of these, 26 had a positive PET/CT for a potential primary tumor site. A second EUA was performed in 17 of these 26 patients and PET/CT-guided biopsy identified 13 primary tumors. In a review by Wong and colleagues,[12] 46 of 78 patients had FDG uptake on PET/CT suspicious of an occult primary cancer. Further investigation confirmed a primary site in 30 of the 46 patients. Overall, PET/CT increased the detection of primary tumor by 38.5%, with a sensitivity, specificity, positive predictive value, and negative predictive value of 100%, 67%, 65%, and 100%, respectively. In 58 patients who had PET/CT scanning after negative EUA and biopsies, 28 had uptake suspicious for a primary site. A second EUA and PET/CT-directed biopsy confirmed a primary site in 16 of these 28 patients.

PET Versus PET/CT Results

Several investigators have compared PET and PET/CT imaging for patients with HNCUP.[19,24] Waltonen and colleagues[19] performed a retrospective study of 183 patients with HNCUP seen over a 10-year period who underwent various imaging modalities. PET was done in 41 patients and identified 14 possible primary tumor sites. Subsequent biopsies confirmed 6 of these 14 sites. Overall, PET scans detected the primary tumor sites in 6 (15%) of 41 patients. PET/CT performed in 52 patients identified 30 possible primary tumor sites. The location of the primary tumor site was confirmed in 23 of these 30 lesions during subsequent endoscopy. In total, PET/CT detected 23

(44%) primary tumors in 52 patients. Those wh[o] had PET/CT had much higher primary tum[or] detection rate than those who did not.

Keller and colleagues[24] reviewed 77 patient[s] with HNCUP who presented from January 200[0] to September 2008. The first 39 consecutiv[e] patients underwent PET scan, and the latter 3[8] patients had PET/CT. PET scan alone had a sens[i]tivity, specificity, positive predictive value, an[d] negative predictive value of 60%, 76%, 46%[,] and 85%, respectively. PET/CT had a sensitivit[y] specificity, positive predictive value, and negativ[e] predictive value of 78%, 95%, 93%, and 83%[,] respectively. PET/CT detected significantly mor[e] primary tumors than PET alone (55% vs 31%[,] $P = .039$). Positive predictive value was signif[i]cantly better in PET/CT than PET (93% vs 46%[,] $P = .01$), and specificity showed a trend towar[d] significance (95% vs 76%, $P = .118$).

Limitations of FDG-PET in HNCUP

Although metabolic imaging can be very helpful i[n] identifying primary tumors in HNCUP, it has som[e] limitations. These include a high false-positive rat[e] in certain situations and limited spatial resolutio[n] leading to a substantial false-negative rate.

Although many primary tumors in HNCUP ar[e] identified in the oropharynx, the reported accurac[y] of FDG-PET in detecting cancers in this region i[s] variable. The lymphatic tissue of Waldeyer rin[g] commonly has a higher level of metabolic activit[y] than other tissues in the head and neck owing t[o] acute and chronic inflammation. This problem i[s] illustrated by the high number of false-positiv[e] PET findings in the tonsil and tongue base. Ther[e] is also physiologic activity from swallowing, saliva[ry] production, speech, and respiration. Patients ar[e] usually instructed to refrain from eating and unnec[-] essary movement while waiting for PET scanning[,] but there is still some appreciable activity that lead[s] to false-positive results[23] (detailed discussion o[f] pitfalls and artifacts in PET scans are discusse[d] elsewhere in this issue by Mehta and colleagues)[.] Biopsy-induced inflammation can potentiall[y] contribute to false-positive results if PET is ob[-] tained after biopsy (see later in this article).

In a retrospective review of 46 patients treated fo[r] occult tonsillar cancer, 6 of the 46 patients under[-] went PET/CT before surgery.[36] Only 1 of the 6 scan[s] correctly identified the tumor, which was actuall[y] a lymphoma. Rusthoven and colleagues' 200[4] review of 16 retrospective studies reported an over[-] all low specificity of PET scan in the palatine tonsil[s] as well as lower sensitivity in the tongue base.[34]

There are also false-negative PET findings a[s] a result of the limited spatial resolution of PE[T] scans. PET resolution is estimated to be about mm.[37,38] Most false-negative PET findings occur with microscopic disease rather than a failure to identify large tumors. One study reported 4 false-negative PET scans with histologically proven tumors.[32] These tumors were in the tonsils and tongue base and had diameters of 0.8 mm to 5.0 m. All of the larger tumors in this study were DG-avid on PET images.

iming to Obtain PET

ecause FDG-PET detects increased metabolic ctivity, inflammation induced by biopsies may ontribute to false-positive results if PET is obtained after biopsy. In the DAHANCA-13 study, ET was performed either before (19/60 patients) r after (41/60 patients) panendoscopy.[30] A false-positive result was found in 1 (12.5%) of 8 atients in the preendoscopy group, compared ith 11 (50%) of 22 patients in the postendoscopy roup. In a retrospective study of 78 patients by Vong and colleagues,[12] 12 (21%) of 58 patients ho had PET/CT after EUA had false-positive esults versus 3 (15%) of 20 false-positive scans those who had PET/CT before EUA. Furthernore, it is not clear how long it is necessary to ait after EUA to reduce the incidence of falseositive PET, as the increased false-positive rate as observed even 5 weeks after biopsy.[23,30]

In addition to reducing false positives, PET obtained before EUA and biopsy can be used to direct iopsy to any suspicious areas. Rudmik and olleagues[25] have shown that PET/CT-directed

biopsy had a significant advantage over the traditional biopsy approach, being able to identify a primary tumor in an additional 30% of patients. Wartski and colleagues[35] were able to identify 13 primary tumors with a second EUA and PET/CT-guided biopsy. All these patients had negative EUA and biopsy by conventional approach before PET/CT scanning. In these cases, patients may have been spared a second surgical endoscopy if PET/CT had been obtained preoperatively.

Although many studies support the idea of obtaining FDG-PET before panendoscopy, this may not be necessary in all cases. As mentioned earlier, 90% of primary tumors are identified by conventional workup. A substantial number of lesions will be identified on operative panendoscopy without needing PET imaging. Also, PET scan can be used by radiation oncologists to assist in treatment planning. If FDG-PET is obtained too early, radiation oncologists may be unable to use it for their purposes. Therefore, the decision of if and when to order FDG-PET should be made by the multidisciplinary cancer treatment team.

IMPACT ON TREATMENT

The most important question to consider is if and how the use of PET in patients with HNCUP results in a change in management. The radiation portal for patients with HNCUP typically includes bilateral necks and the whole pharyngeal axis to cover any potential mucosal sites. If a primary site can be identified, the radiation portal can be reduced and tailored to that specific for the primary tumor site (Fig. 4). Thus, patients might be spared from

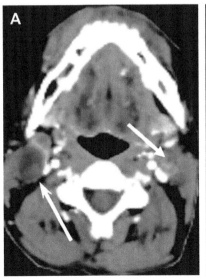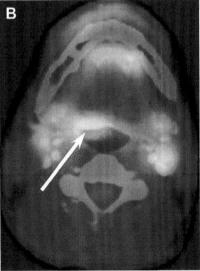

ig. 4. A patient who presented with bilateral level II cervical lymphadenopathy. (A) CT showing bilateral necrotic ymph nodes (arrows). (B) PET/CT showing FDG uptake in the right base of tongue suspicious for the primary umor (arrow). This is not evident on the CT.

extensive radiation therapy and its associated side effects.[39] Detection of previously unknown distant metastases may cause a change from curative to palliative treatment. Some studies report no change in management attributable to PET findings,[11,40] whereas others report changes in treatment in 10% to 60% of patients with HNCUP.[19,28,33,35]

In a review of 16 HNCUP studies, a change in management occurred as a result of PET findings in 37 (24.7%) of 150 patients in the 6 studies that reported these data.[34] In DAHANCA-13, Johansen and colleagues[30] reported a therapeutic change in 15 of 18 patients with true positive PET findings, representing 25% of the studied population (15/60). Of these 15 patients, 10 had radiation volumes changed because of identification of a primary tumor, 4 had no treatment or palliative treatment because of the discovery of extensive metastatic disease, and 1 had surgery for rectal cancer. An estimated 29% change in management was noted from 285 studies evaluating PET for CUP throughout the entire body.[9] In HNCUP, there is an estimated 33% change attributable to PET based on the results of 15 studies.[9]

Interestingly, some investigators changed treatment based on a positive PET finding even without further histologic confirmation, which was done by targeting the radiation fields to the FDG-avid sites.[33,35] This should be done with caution, considering the significant number of false-positive PET findings discussed earlier.

SUMMARY

Identification of the primary tumor is a key goal in the management of HNCUP. FDG-PET, and particularly PET/CT, is a useful imaging modality in the workup of HNCUP, allowing detection of an additional 25% to 30% of primary tumors that are missed by the conventional workup. It can also detect distant metastases that may be otherwise missed. This leads to a change in therapeutic approaches in these patients. Obtaining FDG-PET before EUA and biopsies may reduce the false positives related to biopsy-induced inflammation. Several studies show that PET-directed biopsy is more effective than traditional random biopsies in the detection of the occult primary tumor. However, not all patients require PET imaging to identify a primary tumor. The decision of when and if to obtain a PET scan should be made by the multidisciplinary treatment team.

Although FDG-PET is useful in the workup for HNCUP, it has a high false-positive rate owing to inflammation and physiologic activity in the head and neck, especially in the oropharynx. It also has limited spatial resolution, so is unable to detect very small tumors. Therefore, one must be cautious

in interpreting PET results. A negative PET study patients with HNCUP does not preclude the nee for panendoscopy with biopsy to detect the occu primary tumor. In fact, regardless of the PET PET/CT findings, careful panendoscopy ar directed biopsies should still be performed obtain pathologic confirmation and identify thos tumors that could not be detected by PE Currently, integrated PET/MRI is under develop ment and may soon be used in the clinical settin It will be interesting to see if PET/MRI is superior PET/CT in detecting occult tumors in HNCUP.

REFERENCES

1. Cashman EC, MacMahon PJ, Shelly MJ, et al. Ro of positron emission tomography–computed tomog raphy in head and neck cancer. Ann Otol Rhinol La yngol 2011;120:593–602.
2. van de Wouw AJ, Janssen-Heijnen ML, Coebergh JW et al. Epidemiology of unknown primary tumours; inc dence and population-based survival of 128 patients in Southeast Netherlands, 1984–1992. Eur Cancer 2002;38:409–13.
3. Pavlidis N, Fizazi K. Carcinoma of unknown prima (CUP). Crit Rev Oncol Hematol 2009;69:271–8.
4. Delgado-Bolton RC, Fernández-Pérez C, Gonzále Maté A, et al. Meta-analysis of the performance 18F-FDG PET in primary tumor detection in unknow primary tumors. J Nucl Med 2003;44:1301–14.
5. Fencl P, Belohlavek O, Skopalova M, et al. Prog nostic and diagnostic accuracy of [18F]FDG-PE CT in 190 patients with carcinoma of unknow primary. Eur J Nucl Med Mol Imaging 2007;3 1783–92.
6. Grau C, Johansen LV, Jakobsen J, et al. Cervic lymph node metastases from unknown primar tumours. Results from a national survey by th Danish Society for Head and Neck Oncology. Radic ther Oncol 2000;55:121–9.
7. Nieder C, Gregoire V, Ang KK. Cervical lymph nod metastases from occult squamous cell carcinoma cut down a tree to get an apple? Int J Radiat Onc Biol Phys 2001;50:727–33.
8. Freudenberg LS, Rosenbaum-Krumme SJ, Bockisch A et al. Cancer of unknown primary. Recent Resul Cancer Res 2008;170:193–202.
9. Gambhir SS, Czernin J, Schwimmer J, et a A tabulated summary of the FDG PET literature J Nucl Med 2001;42:1S–93S.
10. Jemal A, Siegel R, Xu J, et al. Cancer statistics 2010. CA Cancer J Clin 2010;60:277–300.
11. Cianchetti M, Mancuso AA, Amdur RJ, et al. Diag nostic evaluation of squamous cell carcinoma meta static to cervical lymph nodes from an unknow head and neck primary site. Laryngoscope 2009 119:2348–54.

22. Wong WL, Sonoda LI, Gharpurhy A, et al. 18F-fluoro-deoxyglucose positron emission tomography/computed tomography in the assessment of occult primary head and neck cancers—an audit and review of published studies. Clin Oncol (R Coll Radiol) 2012;24:190–5.

23. Roh JL, Kim JS, Lee JH, et al. Utility of combined (18)F-fluorodeoxyglucose-positron emission tomography and computed tomography in patients with cervical metastases from unknown primary tumors. Oral Oncol 2009;45:218–24.

24. Hu YY, Liang PY, Lin XP, et al. 18F-FDG PET/CT for the detection of primary tumors metastasizing to lymph nodes of the neck. Ai Zheng 2009;28:312–7 [in Chinese].

25. Medina JE. A rational classification of neck dissections. Otolaryngol Head Neck Surg 1989;100:169–76.

26. Strojan P, Ferlito A, Medina JE, et al. Contemporary management of lymph node metastases from an unknown primary to the neck: I. A review of diagnostic approaches. Head Neck 2011. [Epub ahead of print].

27. Som PM, Curtin HD, Mancuso AA. An imaging-based classification for the cervical nodes designed as an adjunct to recent clinically based nodal classifications. Arch Otolaryngol Head Neck Surg 1999;125:388–96.

28. Grau C. Cervical lymph node metastases from unknown primary tumors. In: Harari PM, Connor NP, Grau C, editors. Functional preservation and quality of life in head and neck radiotherapy. Berlin: Springer Verlag; 2009. p. 125–32.

29. Waltonen JD, Ozer E, Hall NC, et al. Metastatic carcinoma of the neck of unknown primary origin: evolution and efficacy of the modern workup. Arch Otolaryngol Head Neck Surg 2009;135:1024–9.

30. Zhang MQ, El-Mofty SK, Davila RM. Detection of human papillomavirus (HPV)-related squamous cell carcinoma cytologically and by in situ hybridization (ISH) in fine needle aspiration (FNA) biopsies of cervical metastasis: a tool for identifying the site of an occult head and neck primary. Cancer 2008;114:118–23.

31. El-Mofty SK, Zhang MQ, Davila RM. Histologic identification of human papillomavirus (HPV)-related squamous cell carcinoma in cervical lymph nodes: a reliable predictor of the site of an occult head and neck primary carcinoma. Head Neck Pathol 2008;2:163–8.

32. Pfister DJ. The NCCN clinical practice guidelines in oncology. Head and Neck Cancers: Version 2011.2. 2011. p. 58–64. Available at: http://www.nccn.org/professionals/physician_gls/PDF/head-and-neck.pdf. Accessed February 12, 2012.

23. Johansen J, Petersen H, Godballe C, et al. FDG-PET/CT for detection of the unknown primary head and neck tumor. Q J Nucl Med Mol Imaging 2011;55:500–8.

24. Keller F, Psychogios G, Linke R, et al. Carcinoma of unknown primary in the head and neck: comparison between positron emission tomography (PET) and PET/CT. Head Neck 2011;33:1569–75.

25. Rudmik L, Lau HY, Matthews TW, et al. Clinical utility of PET/CT in the evaluation of head and neck squamous cell carcinoma with an unknown primary: a prospective clinical trial. Head Neck 2011;33:935–40.

26. Yabuki K, Tsukuda M, Horiuchi C, et al. Role of 18F-FDG PET in detecting primary site in the patient with primary unknown carcinoma. Eur Arch Otorhinolaryngol 2010;267:1785–92.

27. Bailet JW, Abemayor E, Jabour BA, et al. Positron emission tomography: a new, precise imaging modality for detection of primary head and neck tumors and assessment of cervical adenopathy. Laryngoscope 1992;102:281–8.

28. Dandekar MR, Kannan S, Rangarajan V, et al. Utility of PET in unknown primary with cervical metastasis: a retrospective study. Indian J Cancer 2011;48:181–6.

29. Padovani D, Aimoni C, Zucchetta P, et al. 18-FDG PET in the diagnosis of laterocervical metastases from occult carcinoma. Eur Arch Otorhinolaryngol 2009;266:267–71.

30. Johansen J, Buus S, Loft A, et al. Prospective study of 18FDG-PET in the detection and management of patients with lymph node metastases to the neck from an unknown primary tumor. Results from the DAHANCA-13 study. Head Neck 2008;30:471–8.

31. Silva P, Hulse P, Sykes AJ, et al. Should FDG-PET scanning be routinely used for patients with an unknown head and neck squamous primary? J Laryngol Otol 2007;121:149–53.

32. Miller FR, Hussey D, Beeram M, et al. Positron emission tomography in the management of unknown primary head and neck carcinoma. Arch Otolaryngol Head Neck Surg 2005;131:626–9.

33. Wong WL, Saunders M. The impact of FDG PET on the management of occult primary head and neck tumours. Clin Oncol (R Coll Radiol) 2003;15:461–6.

34. Rusthoven KE, Koshy M, Paulino AC. The role of fluorodeoxyglucose positron emission tomography in cervical lymph node metastases from an unknown primary tumor. Cancer 2004;101:2641–9.

35. Wartski M, Le Stanc E, Gontier E, et al. In search of an unknown primary tumour presenting with cervical metastases: performance of hybrid FDG-PET-CT. Nucl Med Commun 2007;28:365–71.

36. Nabili V, Zaia B, Blackwell KE, et al. Positron emission tomography: poor sensitivity for occult tonsillar cancer. Am J Otolaryngol 2007;28:153–7.

37. Salem S, Patel NH, Barwick T, et al. Occult squamous cell carcinoma of the uvula detected by F-18 FDG PET/CT in a case of carcinoma of unknown

primary in the head and neck. Clin Nucl Med 2010; 35:800–1.

38. Braams JW, Pruim J, Kole AC, et al. Detection of unknown primary head and neck tumors by positron emission tomography. Int J Oral Maxillofac Surg 1997;26:112–5.

39. Jereczek-Fossa BA, Jassem J, Orecchia R. Cervical lymph node metastases of squamous cell carcinoma from an unknown primary. Cancer Treat Rev 2004;3 153–64.

40. Deron PB, Bonte KM, Vermeersch HF, et al. Lymp node metastasis of squamous cell carcinoma fro an unknown primary in the upper and middle nec impact of (18)F-fluorodeoxyglucose positron emi sion tomography/computed tomography. Canc Biother Radiopharm 2011;26:331–4.

PET Scan in Thyroid Cancer

Muammer Urhan, MD[a], Sandip Basu, MD[b], Abass Alavi, MD[c],*

KEYWORDS

- PET • Differentiated thyroid carcinoma • ^{18}F-fluorodeoxyglucose • ^{124}I • ^{18}F-DOPA
- ^{68}Ga-DOTATOC

KEY POINTS

- The most widely advocated indication of fluorodeoxyglucose (FDG)-PET in differentiated thyroid cancer is in evaluating patients with high thyroglobulin level when radioiodine whole-body scan is negative.
- FDG-PET imaging can provide prognostic information and thus may be useful in identifying the patients at higher risk of recurrent and metastatic disease.
- The role of novel PET tracers such as 18F-dihydroxyphenylalanine and ^{68}Ga-DOTA-NOC/^{68}Ga-DOTA-TATE in medullary thyroid carcinoma and use of ^{124}I in differentiated thyroid carcinoma (especially for lesional dosimetry) continues to evolve with promising results.

INTRODUCTION

Thyroid cancer is a group of tumors with different histologic and behavioral features including follicular cell–derived papillary thyroid carcinoma (PTC), follicular thyroid carcinoma (FTC), and Hürthle cell thyroid carcinoma (HTC). Medullary thyroid carcinoma (MTC) originates from parafollicular C cells scattered around the follicular epithelium in thyroid gland. Thyroid cancer accounts for approximately 1% to 3% of all cancer cases; however, its incidence has increased significantly around the world in the past 3 decades. The age-adjusted incidence was 11.6 per 100,000 per year. It has been estimated that approximately 56,500 men and women will be diagnosed with thyroid cancer, and about 1800 of them will die of the disease in 2012. PTC comprises most of the thyroid cancer cases (up to 80%) and more than 70% of patients are women. The median age at diagnosis for thyroid cancer was 50 years of age.[1] The risk for developing thyroid cancer increases in patients receiving external beam radiation to the head and neck, especially in

childhood. Also at risk are those who have been irradiated internally following radioactive fallout and those with a family history of thyroid malignancy.[2] The incidence of thyroid cancer and the dose of irradiation have been closely correlated with exposures up to 1500 cGy, but the cancer risk is not increased at higher doses, probably because of the cell death from the radiation. Another factor for developing thyroid cancer is the iodine supply: follicular or anaplastic subtype of thyroid cancer is frequently seen in countries with low iodine intake, whereas there is a tendency to PTC in populations in which dietary iodine ingestion is adequate.

Differentiated thyroid cancer (DTC) has a favorable prognosis with overall 10-year survival rates of about 80% to 93%. However, recurrent disease in the neck may develop in up to 40% of patients, most commonly in the first 2 years following initial treatment with the following risk factors: incomplete surgery, an aggressive histologic subtype (tall cell, columnar cell), age greater than 45 years at initial diagnosis, tumor size more than 4 cm, extrathyroidal extension of the primary tumor, and

[a] Department of Nuclear Medicine, GATA Haydarpasa Training Hospital, Tibbiye Cad, Uskudar, Istanbul 34668, Turkey; [b] Radiation Medicine Centre (BARC), Tata Memorial Hospital Annexe, Jerbai Wadia Road, Parel, Mumbai 400012, India; [c] Division of Nuclear Medicine, Department of Radiology, Hospital of the University of Pennsylvania, 3400 Spruce Street, 110 Donner Building, Philadelphia, PA 19104, USA
* Corresponding author.
E-mail address: alaviabass@yahoo.com

PET Clin 7 (2012) 453–461
http://dx.doi.org/10.1016/j.cpet.2012.06.008
1556-8598/12/$ – see front matter © 2012 Elsevier Inc. All rights reserved.

lymph node involvement.[3] Mortality is about 8% and the underlying cause of death is usually local compression of the trachea and vasculature in the neck.

The thyroid tumors usually retain many of the characteristics of their normal progenitor cells such as iodine avidity, capacity to secrete thyroid hormones, and capacity to synthesize thyroglobulin (Tg). In the surveillance period, radioiodine scanning has been a well-established procedure in detecting recurrent or metastatic disease in patients with differentiated thyroid carcinoma when serum Tg level is increased, but the non–iodine-avid thyroid tumor poses a diagnostic and therapeutic challenge. The persistent tumor should be localized precisely and treated with either surgery or external beam radiation treatment because it will gain no benefit from ^{131}I treatment.[4] However, recurrent or metastatic tumor is seldom localized precisely with anatomic imaging modalities including ultrasound, computerized tomography (CT), and magnetic resonance (MR) imaging. In particular, ultrasound of the neck is useful for detecting small cervical adenopathy; however, it is often inconclusive in discriminating between malignant lesions and nonspecific tissue changes in the postsurgical neck.

FLUORODEOXYGLUCOSE-PET AND PET/CT SCAN IN PATIENTS WITH DIFFERENTIATED THYROID CARCINOMA

Radioiodine whole-body scanning (WBS) has been well established in the management of patients with thyroid carcinoma provided that the original tumor cells are well differentiated and have the ability to concentrate radioiodine. However, in up to 30% of patients with differentiated thyroid carcinoma, tumor cells lose the ability to take up radioiodine, which impairs the clinical role of iodine isotopes and limits their use for diagnostic and therapeutic purposes.

Metabolic imaging with PET using [^{18}F]fluorodeoxyglucose (^{18}F-FDG) seems to be a valuable diagnostic tool in patients with non–iodine-avid thyroid tumor, particularly in the setting of high and gradually increasing Tg levels (Fig. 1). An ^{18}F-FDG-PET scan provides unique metabolic information and complements anatomic imaging findings in the characterization of non–iodine-avid thyroid tumor and leads the patients to alternative treatments including surgical intervention and external beam radiation. In a multicenter trial by Grünwald and colleagues,[5] the sensitivity of FDG-PET was 75% in the whole group and 85% in the subgroup of patients with negative ^{131}I WBS. Integrated PET/CT or PET/MR imaging devices provides additional structural information

in the same session that helps in discriminating persistent or recurrent thyroid cancer from nonspecific FDG uptake in the neck and improve the diagnosis of persistent or recurrent thyroid cancer.[6–9]

FDG-PET has been most useful in patients with poorly differentiated or anaplastic thyroid carcinoma, which are known to have increased glucose metabolism and limited or no radioiodine uptake (Fig. 2). More than 80% of patients with HTC have negative radioiodine scanning, whereas FDG uptake by tumor cells has been reported to be high. It is more aggressive than other types of DTC and has a worse prognosis, especially when the primary tumor is widely invasive. HTC has higher incidence of distant metastasis, and cervical lymph node metastasis is frequent at initial diagnosis. The combination of serum Tg measurement and radioiodine WBS is used for the detection of recurrent or metastatic HTC, but the sensitivity of diagnostic radioiodine scanning has been as low as 18%.[10] Accurate localization of the disease site is essential; surgical intervention and external beam radiation treatment are the only options for cure because non–iodine-avid tumor cells do not benefit from high-dose radioiodine treatment. PET scanning often provides additional information compared with conventional imaging and contributes to localizing the tumor in patients with a clinical suspicion of recurrent or metastatic tumor because of increasing Tg levels. FDG-PET has a sensitivity, specificity, and accuracy of 92%, 80%, and 89%, respectively, reported in a meta-analysis by Plotkin and colleagues.[11] If the tumor secretes no Tg, which is an important marker for early detection of recurrent and metastatic thyroid cancer, FDG-PET remains the only diagnostic tool to diagnose persistent disease after initial thyroidectomy. Furthermore, thyroid tumors contain both differentiated and undifferentiated tumor cells, so FDG-PET should not be limited to only ^{131}I WBS negative patients. The accuracy of FDG-PET scan increases when it is used together with ^{131}I scanning. Using this combination, tumor sites were missed in only 7% of all thyroid cancer cases.[12,13]

It has been postulated that cellular metabolism is stimulated with recombinant thyroid-stimulating hormone (TSH) (rhTSH) and thus more FDG is accumulated inside the thyroid cancer cells. Some investigators suggested that the sensitivity of FDG-PET is higher when it is performed under TSH stimulation (rhTSH) compared with TSH suppression, and that more FDG-avid lesions are detected because of better resolution of the PET instrument. However, some investigators reported no significant impact of TSH stimulation on scan interpretation.[14,15] The potential benefits and the

A   **B**

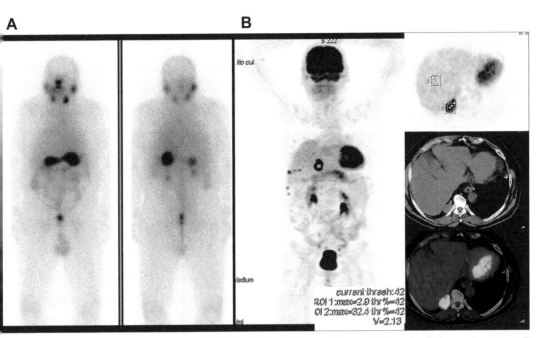

ig. 1. Negative I-131 posttreatment scan with 200 mCi in a 66-year-old man with gradually increasing serum Tg
vels (initially 38 ng/dL, later 800 ng/dL within a period of 4 months) (*A*). Multiple lesions at the lower part of the
ght lung with high glucose metabolism rates (SUV_{max}, 32.4) were clearly defined on FDG-PET scan (*B*).

ost of the agent should be taken into account,
articularly in patients with suspected recurrent
yroid cancer and negative iodine scan findings.

HE PROGNOSTIC ROLE OF FDG-PET IN HYROID CANCER

he overall prognosis in thyroid carcinoma is vari-
ble; the 10-year survival rates for patients with
apillary, follicular, Hürthle cell and anaplastic
yroid cancer are about 93%, 85%, 76%, and
4% respectively. Radioiodine uptake by the
mor cells, the age at initial diagnosis, extrathyroi-
al extension, gender, and grade and histology of
ne tumor (subtype, grade, and size) are the major
rognostic factors that help to stratify the patient
to high-risk and low-risk groups. Iodine avidity
eflects a differentiated form of thyroid cancer,
vhereas non–iodine-avid thyroid tumor with high
lucose metabolism is usually associated with
 more aggressive clinical course. FDG-PET
naging has been useful in providing prognostic
nformation and determining whether patients are
t higher risk of the recurrent and metastatic
isease. Thus the low-risk patients should not be
reated with therapies that may have long-term
ide effects. The prognosis of the patients with
DG-avid lesions is poor. Their survivals are
nversely proportional to the volume of the disease
nd were found to have a significant correlation

with the maximum standardized uptake value
(SUV), suggesting that, in thyroid tumor, the higher
the metabolic activity, the more aggressive the
disease. Although Tg secretion is a marker of
good differentiation, the potential for a positive
PET scan becomes greater when serum Tg value
is increased. FDG-PET detected the tumor site in
11%, 50%, and 93% of patients with serum Tg
levels of less than 10, 10 to 20, and greater than
100 µg/L, respectively.[16]

The prognostic information provided by FDG-
PET contributes significantly to decision making
for local or systemic therapy and the use of alternative methods such as retinoic acids to improve
the differentiation of the lesions for subsequent
use of ^{131}I for therapeutic purposes.[17]

EVALUATION FDG UPTAKE IN THE THYROID

The normal thyroid gland takes up little or no FDG;
however, on PET scans, incidental increased FDG
uptake in thyroid has been reported in 1.8% to
2.9% of all patients. The role of FDG-PET scan in
the investigation of thyroid lesions and differentiating between benign and malignant nodules is
controversial. When the uptake is diffuse inside
the thyroid gland, the incidence of malignancy is
low. Such uptake is often caused by lymphocytes
in Hashimoto disease or by hypermetabolic thyro-
cytes in Graves disease. However, in patients with

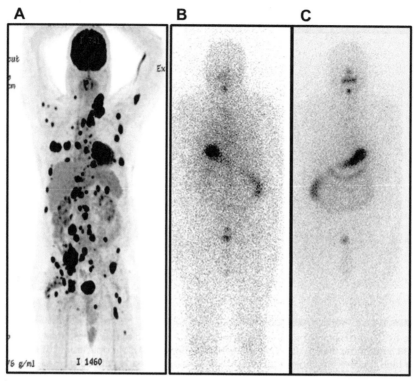

Fig. 2. Multiple metastatic lesions on FDG-PET scan in a 72-year-old man with papillary carcinoma (A). On whole body scan, no lesion was iodine avid except the residual thyroid tissue in the neck (B, C).

thyroid lymphoma and widespread infiltration of thyroid gland by metastatic tumors, similar findings may be seen on PET images.[18–21] Focal FDG uptake has been associated with thyroid cancer in approximately 30% to 50% of patients, which is greater than the 4% to 12.6% risk in thyroid nodules detected by ultrasound (**Fig. 3**). The contribution of SUV measurement in differentiating the malignancy from benign lesions has been equivocal. Some investigators suggested that SUV is valuable in this respect, whereas others reported overlapping values and no significant difference between the benign and malignant thyroid lesions. The range in SUV of the malignant and benign lesions is attributed to several factors including the partial volume effect, high FDG uptake in some benign lesions such as Hürthle cell and autonomous adenoma, hyperthyroidism, TSH levels, inflammation, and the presence of well-differentiated (iodine-avid) thyroid cancer cells.[22,23]

THE ROLE OF ^{124}I PET IN DIFFERENTIATED THYROID CARCINOMA

Radioactive iodine imaging for thyroid cancer is imaging iodine transportation by the sodium iodine transporters that are present in about 80% of DTC

cells. ^{124}I is a PET agent with physical half-life of 4.2 days. It disintegrates by producing positrons of high energies (1532 keV and 2135 keV), high energy γ and x-rays, and provides high-resolution quantitative imaging data. Because ^{131}I is the main agent for treatment, ^{124}I can be used as a surrogate in patients with DTC before therapeutic interventions.

The acquisition of PET images seems to be feasible using a bismuth germanate (BGO)–based PET scanner in three-dimensional (3D) mode with narrow energy window. It has been preferred to the conventional two-dimensional (2D) mode because of downscatter of high-energy photons in the lead or tungsten septa. Newer PET systems using lutetium oxyorthosilicate (LSO) with narrow energy and coincidence-timing window have advantages compared with BGO scanners.[24] ^{124}I PET offers high-resolution images and provides specific dosimetric information and quantification of the volume of the thyroid tumor. Although the main purpose of ^{124}I PET scan is lesion dosimetry, these findings reveal that ^{124}I PET/CT may be useful for providing additional diagnostic information. The introduction of hybrid imaging (PET/CT) has improved the lesion detection rates from 87% to 100% for ^{124}I PET alone and ^{124}I PET/CT scan, respectively.[25–27]

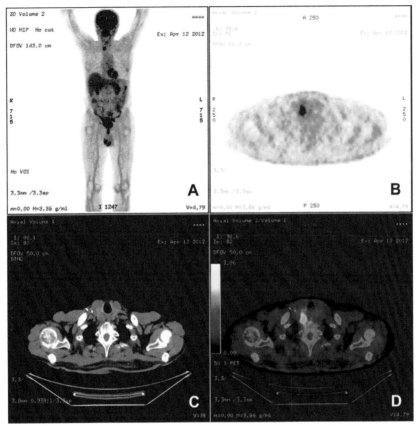

Fig. 3. FDG-PET/CT maximum-intensity projection (MIP) (*A*) and transaxial scans (*B*, PET; *C*, CT; *D*, fused) of 58-year-old man with pancreatic cancer. A focal FDG uptake was noted in the inferior pole of the right thyroid lobe (SUV$_{max}$, 6.9) and the lesion was proved to be papillary thyroid cancer by histopathology.

[124]I PET dosimetry has changed patient management in 25% of cases in terms of determining the therapeutic dose of ^{131}I administered, and led to early multimodality intervention in 32% of patients.[28] However, the use of [124]I PET dosimetry in routine clinical practice is still limited by availability and the cost of [124]I.

PET SCAN IN MTC

MTC has similar histologic features to other neuroendocrine tumors such as carcinoid and islet cell tumors. It is often sporadic but there might be familial cases as a part of multiple endocrine neoplasia syndromes type 2 (MEN2). The prognosis is associated with the extent of the primary tumor: the overall 10-year survival rates are 90% when the primary tumor is confined to the thyroid gland, and 70% and 20% in the presence of cervical lymph node metastases and spread to distant organ, respectively. MTC is treated with thyroidectomy. For surveillance, patients are traditionally monitored with determination of serum calcitonin. In patients with gradually increasing serum calcitonin levels, the thyroid bed and the neck should be investigated initially with either ultrasound, CT, or MR imaging for locoregional recurrence of the tumor, because surgical intervention is the only option.

FDG-PET scan is promising and more sensitive than anatomic imaging and functional imaging using single-photon emission tracers in detecting recurrent and metastatic tumors in patients with MTC. It was particularly useful for determination of cervical lymph node metastases, detecting more cervical, supraclavicular, and mediastinal lesions compared with anatomic imaging methods.[29,30] In one of the early reports, de Groot and colleagues[31] observed that ^{18}F-FDG-PET detected more lesions than [99m]technetium (^{99m}Tc) dimercaptosuccinic acid (V) and ^{111}In-labeled octreotide, as well as bone scintigraphy combined with anatomic imaging such as ultrasound, CT, or MR imaging. Rubello and colleagues[32] evaluated 19 patients with MTC with increased serum calcitonin levels (58–1350 pg/mL) and reported that ^{18}F-FDG-PET/CT was an accurate imaging modality in detecting metastases in patients with recurrent MTC with increased serum calcitonin levels.

However, unlike DTC cells, it has been reported that there was no increase in expression of the glucose transporter proteins GLUT 1 to GLUT 5 in MTC cells.[33] This may explain the decreased ^{18}F-FDG avidity in persistent tumors and false-negative PET studies in patients with high serum calcitonin levels. The size of the lesion is another factor because small tumor volume can also lead to false-negative PET scans. Therefore, although hybrid imaging with CT improved the diagnostic accuracy of PET in detection of recurrent and metastatic MTC, the role of ^{18}F-FDG-PET in MTC has been questioned by some investigators regarding its limited role in neuroendocrine tumors (NETs). MTC has certain features of neuroendocrine tumors, such as the presence of amine uptake mechanisms and/or peptide receptors at the cell membrane, allowing the clinical use of specific radiopharmaceuticals to reflect the metabolism of the tumor cells, as discussed later.

NOVEL PET AGENTS IN THYROID CANCER

In the last decade, along with increasing use of PET systems, novel non-FDG-PET agents have been widely investigated in oncology. Among them, ^{18}F-dihydroxyphenylalanine, (^{18}F-DOPA) and ^{18}F-fluorodopamine (^{18}F-FDA) have been shown to be promising for evaluation of patients with MTC. In particular, the results obtained from ^{18}F-DOPA studies are noteworthy.[34,35] L-DOPA is a precursor of catecholamine metabolism and is converted to dopamine by the aromatic amino acid decarboxylase (AADC) enzymes. Hoeger and colleagues[35] reported that the sensitivity ^{18}F-DOPA-PET was 63%, which was lower than that of CT/MR imaging but better than those of ^{18}F-FDG-PET and ultrasound. In a retrospective analysis of ^{18}F-DOPA-PET in 15 patients with MTC who had increased levels of tumor marker Beuthien-Baumann and colleagues[36] found similar results for ^{18}F-FDG and ^{18}F-DOPA.

Somatostatin analogues have recently been labeled with various positron emitters such as gallium-68 (^{68}Ga) and copper-64 (^{64}Cu). [68]Ga a generator-produced radionuclide that can be chelated with DOTA to form a stable [^{68}Ga-DOTA Tyr3] octreotide complex (^{68}Ga-DOTATOC). Other ^{68}Ga labeled somatostatin analogues have consequently been developed, including ^{68}Ga-DOTA NOC, by replacing the C-terminal threoninol DOTATOC with threonine, and [^{68}Ga-DOTA Tyr3] octreotate (^{68}Ga-DOTA-TATE).[37–39] Imaging is principally based on binding to the somatostatin receptors that are found on normal tissues, including those of the central nervous system, anterior pituitary, thyroid, pancreas, gastrointestinal tract, spleen, and adrenals, but that are overexpressed on tumor cells originating from these organ systems.[40,41] This is particularly important for detection of persistent non–iodine-avid thyroid tumors that have little FDG uptake (**Fig. 4**). After successful tumor delineation with ^{68}Ga-DOTA complexes, the next step was peptide receptor radionuclide treatment with somatostatin analogues labeled with high-energy β-emitters including yttrium-90 (^{90}Y) and lutetium-177 ([177]Lu

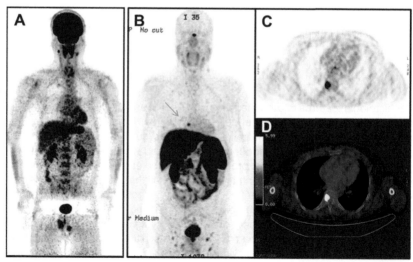

Fig. 4. Non–FDG-avid metastatic lesion in thoracic-8 vertebral body (*A*) was seen on Ga-68 DOTATOC PET scan MIP (*B; arrow*); (*C*) transaxial PET; (*D*) fused.

patients who had inoperable and/or metasta-zed tumor.[42,43]

ET SCAN IN DETECTING LOCOREGIONAL HYROID CANCER IN THE NECK

ersistent disease or lymph node metastases ave been reported in 36% to 40% of patients ith thyroid cancer (especially with papillary and nedullary forms) in which lymphatic infiltration is ne main mode of spread.[44] The presence of nyroid capsule extension and soft tissue invasion the thyroid bed or lymph node metastasis has worse prognosis for survival in patients with nyroid cancer and may affect patient manage-nent. It is essential to remove all clinically evident nvolved lymph nodes by surgery, if possible. After urgery, the efficacy of subsequent high-dose ra-ioiodine treatment to ablate microscopic disease nproves and the accuracy of monitoring post-reatment serum Tg levels increases significantly. Vhole-body PET scan is the most useful imaging nodality for accurate detection of neck nodal isease and exclusion of distant metastasis, thus acilitating selection of patients for surgery (Fig. 5).

After initial treatment, periodic serum Tg mea-urement and diagnostic low-dose radioiodine canning have been well-established methods for creening recurrent or metastatic thyroid cancer. Iowever, inconsistent results have been obtained in approximately one-third of patients with recur-rent neck disease, indicating that these 2 methods cannot be relied on to detect neck lesions accu-rately. Characterization of lymph nodes with CT or MR imaging is primarily based on size criteria and therefore both imaging modalities have false-negative rates ranging from 10% to 30%. PET has proved to be beneficial in ambiguous cases even in patients with normal-sized neck lymph nodes, especially in those with intermediate-risk to high-risk features.[45] Debates are ongoing concerning the capability of PET in detecting small cervical lymph nodes. The potential reasons for false-negative PET scans include small tumor burden, cystic degeneration of metastatic nodes (fre-quently seen in PTC), and decreased tracer uptake by metastatic nodes with a low metabolic rate.[9,16] In the clinical setting, ultrasound of the anterior and lateral neck is usually the first-line diagnostic method for assessing persistent thyroid tumor or cervical lymph node metastasis. Ultrasound-guided fine-needle aspiration has a true-positive rate of 95.3% and the cost of the procedure is low. PET scan seems to be superior to other func-tional or anatomic imaging methods (eg, ^{201}Tl and ^{99m}Tc-sestamibi, CT, MR imaging), especially in detecting small metastatic deposits in the neck. However, it should be used as a complementary method, rather than a counterpart to ultrasound, CT, or MR imaging in the surveillance of patients

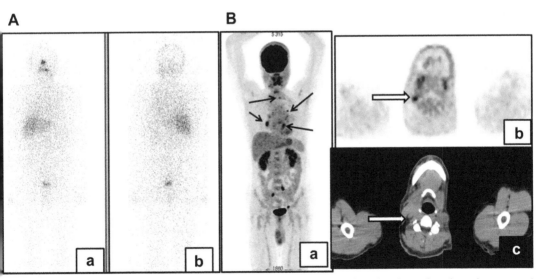

Fig. 5. A 52-year-old man with papillary thyroid cancer had right lateral neck solitary lymph node metastasis onfirmed by ultrasound-guided fine needle aspiration biopsy. Serum Tg level was 87 ng/dL and I-131 whole-ody diagnostic scan with 5 mCi was negative (Aa, b). The patient had FDG-PET scan (Ba–c) because of inappro-riately high serum Tg levels, and additional metastatic lesions were revealed on PET scan in upper mediastinum, ilateral hilar, and mediastinal regions (arrows). The initial plan was to perform modified right neck dissection; iowever, it was altered after detecting multiple additional lesions with FDG-PET scan and the patient was eferred to external beam radiation treatment.

with thyroid cancer in the presence of negative radioiodine scanning and normal serum Tg levels.[13,46]

REFERENCES

1. Howlader N, Noone AM, Krapcho M, et al. editors. SEER Cancer Statistics Review, 1975-2009 (Vintage 2009 populations), National Cancer Institute. Bethesda (MD). Available at: http://seer.cancer.gov/csr/1975_pops09/. based on November 2011 SEER data submission, posted to the SEER web site, 2012. Accessed August 3, 2012.

2. Pacini F, Castagna MG, Cipri C, et al. Medullary thyroid carcinoma. Clin Oncol (R Coll Radiol) 2010; 22:475–85.

3. Mazzaferri EL. An overview of the management of thyroid cancer. In: Mazzaferri EL, Harmer C, Mallick UK, et al, editors. Practical management of thyroid cancer: a multidisciplinary approach. London: Springer-Verlag; 2006. p. 1–8.

4. Mian C, Barollo S, Pennelli G, et al. Molecular characteristics in papillary thyroid cancers (PTCs) with no ^{131}I uptake. Clin Endocrinol 2008;68:108–16.

5. Grunwald F, Kalicke T, Feine U, et al. Fluorine-18 fluorodeoxyglucose positron emission tomography in thyroid cancer: results of a multicentre study. Eur J Nucl Med 1999;26:1547–52.

6. McDougal IR, Davidson J, Segall SM. Positron emission tomography of the thyroid, with an emphasis on thyroid cancer. Nucl Med Commun 2001;22:485–92.

7. Iagaru A, Kalinyak JE, McDougall IR. F-18 FDG PET/CT in the management of thyroid cancer. Clin Nucl Med 2007;32:690–5.

8. Zoller M, Kohlfuerst S, Igerc I, et al. Combined PET/CT in the follow-up of differentiated thyroid carcinoma: what is the impact of each modality? Eur J Nucl Med Mol Imaging 2007;34:487–95.

9. Yeo JS, Chung JK, So Y, et al. F-18-fluoro-deoxyglucose positron emission tomography as a presurgical evaluation modality for I-131 negative thyroid carcinoma patients with local recurrence in cervical lymph nodes. Head Neck 2001;23:94–103.

10. Yen TC, Lin HD, Lee CH, et al. The role of technetium-99m sestamibi whole-body scan in diagnosing metastatic hurtle cell carcinoma of thyroid gland after total thyroidectomy: a comparison with iodine-131 and thalium-201 whole-body scans. Eur J Nucl Med 1994;21:980–3.

11. Plotkin M, Hautzel H, Krause BJ, et al. Implication of 2-(18)fluor-2-deoxyglucose positron emission tomography in the follow-up of Hürthle cell thyroid cancer. Thyroid 2002;12:155–61.

12. Feine U, Lietzenmayer R, Hanke JP, et al. Fluorine-18-FDG and iodine-131-iodide uptake in thyroid cancer. J Nucl Med 1996;37:1468–72.

13. Grünwald F, Menzel C, Bender H, et al. Comparison of [18]FDG-PET with [131]iodine and ^{99m}Tc-sestamibi scintigraphy in differentiated thyroid cancer. Thyroid 1997;7:327–35.

14. van Tol KM, Jager PL, Piers DA, et al. Better yield of (18)fluorodeoxyglucose-positron emission tomography in patients with metastatic differentiated thyroid carcinoma during thyrotropin stimulation. Thyroid 2002;12(5):381–7.

15. Chin BB, Patel P, Cohade C, et al. Recombinant human thyrotropin stimulation of fluoro-D-glucose positron emission tomography uptake in well differentiated thyroid carcinoma. J Clin Endocrine Metab 2004;89(1):91–5.

16. Wang W, Macapinlac H, Larson SM, et al. [18F]-2-fluoro-2-deoxy-D-glucose positron emission tomography localizes residual thyroid cancer in patients with negative diagnostic ([131])I whole body scan and elevated serum thyroglobulin levels. J Clin Endocrinol Metab 1999;84:2291–302.

17. Schluter B, Bohuslavizki KH, Beyer W, et al. Impact of FDG PET on patients with differentiated thyroid cancer who present with elevated thyroglobulin and negative ^{131}I scan. J Nucl Med 2001;42:71–6.

18. Boerner AR, Voth E, Theissen P, et al. Glucose metabolism of the thyroid in Graves' disease measured by F-18-fluorodeoxyglucose positron emission tomography. Thyroid 1998;8:765–72.

19. Boerner AR, Voth E, Theissen P, et al. Glucose metabolism of the thyroid in autonomous goiter measured by F-18-FDG-PET. Exp Clin Endocrinol Diabetes 2000;108:191–6.

20. Karantanis D, Bogsrud TV, Wiseman GA, et al. Clinical significance of diffusely increased 18F-FDG uptake in the thyroid gland. J Nucl Med 2007;48:896–901.

21. Deandreis D, Al Ghuzlan A, Auperin A, et al. Is 1-F-fluorodeoxyglucose PET/CT useful for the presurgical characterization of thyroid nodules with indeterminate fine needle aspiration cytology? Thyroid 2012;22(2):165.

22. Burguera B, Gharib H. Thyroid incidentalomas: prevalence, diagnosis, significance, and management. Endocrinol Metab Clin North Am 2000;29: 187–203.

23. Geus-Oei LF, Pieters GF, Bonenkamp JJ, et al. 18FFDG PET reduces unnecessary hemithyroidectomies for thyroid nodules with inconclusive cytologic results. J Nucl Med 2006;47:770–5.

24. Sgouros G, Kolbert KS, Sheikh A, et al. Patient-specific dosimetry for I-131 thyroid cancer therapy using I-124 PET and 3-dimensional-internal dosimetry (3D-ID) software. J Nucl Med 2004;45:1366–72.

25. Pentlow KS, Graham MC, Lambrecht RM, et al. Quantitative imaging of iodine-124 with PET. J Nucl Med 1996;37:1557–62.

26. Rault E, Vandenberghe S, Van Holen R, et al. Comparison of image quality of different iodine

isotopes (I-123, I-124, and I-131). Cancer Biother Radiopharm 2007;22:423–30.

. Eschmann SM, Reischl G, Bilger K, et al. Evaluation of dosimetry of radioiodine therapy in benign and malignant thyroid disorders by means of iodine-124 and PET. Eur J Nucl Med Mol Imaging 2002;29:760–7.

. Freudenberg LS, Jentzen W, Marlowe RJ, et al. 124-Iodine positron emission tomography/computed tomography dosimetry in pediatric patients with differentiated thyroid cancer. Exp Clin Endocrinol Diabetes 2007;115:690–3.

. Brandt-Mainz K, Muller SP, Gorges R, et al. The value of F-18 FDG PET in patients with medullary thyroid cancer. Eur J Nucl Med 2000;27:490–6.

. Szakall S Jr, Esik O, Balzik G, et al. F-18 FDG-PET detection of lymph node metastases in medullary thyroid carcinoma. J Nucl Med 2002;43(1):66–71.

. de Groot JW, Links TP, Jager PL, et al. Impact of F-18 fluoro-2-deoxy-D-glucose positron emission tomography (FDG-PET) in patients with biochemical evidence of recurrent or residual medullary thyroid cancer. Ann Surg Oncol 2004;11(8):786–94.

. Rubello D, Rampin L, Nanni C, et al. The role of ^{18}F-FDG PET/CT in detecting metastatic deposits of recurrent medullary thyroid carcinoma: a prospective study. Eur J Surg Oncol 2007;34(5):581–6.

. Musholt TJ, Musholt PB, Dehdashti F, et al. Evaluation of fluorodeoxyglucose-positron emission tomographic scanning and its association with glucose transporter expression in medullary thyroid carcinoma and pheochromocytoma: a clinical and molecular study. Surgery 1997;122:1049–60.

. Koopmans KP, de Groot JW, Plukker JT, et al. 18F-dihydroxyphenylalanine PET in patients with biochemical evidence of medullary thyroid cancer: relation to tumor differentiation. J Nucl Med 2008;49(4):524–31.

. Hoegerle S, Ghanem N, Altehoefer C, et al. ^{18}F-DOPA positron emission tomography for the detection of glomus tumours. Eur J Nucl Med Mol Imaging 2003;30:689–94.

. Beuthien-Baumann B, Strumpf A, Zessin J, et al. Diagnostic impact of PET with ^{18}F-FDG, 18F-DOPA and 3-O-methyl-6- [18]Ffluoro-DOPA in recurrent or metastatic medullary thyroid carcinoma. Eur J Nucl Med Mol Imaging 2007;34:1604–9.

37. Gabriel M, Decristoforo C, Kendler D, et al. ^{68}Ga-DOTA-Try3-octreotide PET in neuroendocrine tumors: comparison with somatostatin receptor scintigraphy and CT. J Nucl Med 2007;48:508–18.

38. Fanti S, Ambrosini V, Tomassetti P, et al. Evaluation of unusual neuroendocrine tumors by means of ^{68}Ga-DOTA-NOC PET. Biomed Pharmacother 2008; 62:667–71.

39. Krausz Y, Freedman N, Rubinstein R, et al. ^{68}Ga-DOTA-NOC PET/CT imaging of neuroendocrine tumors: comparison with (111)In-DTPA-octreotide(OctreoScan). Mol Imaging Biol 2010;13:583–93.

40. Kwekkeboom DJ, Krenning EP, Sheidhauer K, et al. ENETS Consensus Guidelines for the Standards of Care in Neuroendocrine Tumors: somatostatin receptor imaging with (111)In-pentetreotide. Neuroendocrinology 2009;90:184–9.

41. Reubi JC, Lantold AM. High density of somatostatin receptors in pituitary tumors from acromegalic patients. J Clin Endocrinol Metab 1984;59:1148–51.

42. Bushnell DL Jr, O'Dorisio TM, O'Dorisio MS, et al. 90Y-edotreotide for metastatic carcinoid refractory to octreotide. J Clin Oncol 2010;28:1652–9.

43. Kwekkeboom DJ, de Herder WW, Kam BL, et al. Treatment with the radiolabeled somatostatin analogue [177Lu-DOTA 0, Tyr3]octreotate: toxicity, efficacy, and survival. J Clin Oncol 2008;26:2124–30.

44. Shaha AB, Shah JP, Loree TR. Patterns of nodal and distant metastasis based on histologic varieties in differentiated carcinoma of the thyroid. Am J Surg 1996;172:692–4.

45. Kim MH, O JH, Ko SH, et al. Role of [(18)F]-fluorodeoxy-D-glucose positron emission tomography and computed tomography in the early detection of persistent/recurrent thyroid carcinoma in intermediate-to-high risk patients following initial radioactive iodine ablation therapy. Thyroid 2012;22(2):157–64.

46. Frilling A, Gorges R, Tecklenborg K, et al. Value of preoperative diagnostic modalities in patients with recurrent thyroid carcinoma. Surgery 2000;128: 1067–74.

Index

Note: Page numbers of article titles are in **boldface** type.

PET Clin 7 (2012) 463–465
http://dx.doi.org/10.1016/S1556-8598(12)00113-7
1556-8598/12/$ – see front matter © 2012 Elsevier Inc. All rights reserved.

Moving?

Make sure your subscription moves with you!

To notify us of your new address, find your **Clinics Account Number** (located on your mailing label above your name), and contact customer service at:

Email: journalscustomerservice-usa@elsevier.com

800-654-2452 (subscribers in the U.S. & Canada)
314-447-8871 (subscribers outside of the U.S. & Canada)

Fax number: 314-447-8029

Elsevier Health Sciences Division
Subscription Customer Service
3251 Riverport Lane
Maryland Heights, MO 63043

*To ensure uninterrupted delivery of your subscription, please notify us at least 4 weeks in advance of move.

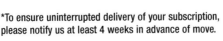

Printed and bound by CPI Group (UK) Ltd, Croydon, CR0 4YY

03/10/2024

01040352-0005